Emergency Communication

Giolo Fele

Emergency Communication

The Organization of Calls to Emergency Dispatch Centers

palgrave
macmillan

Giolo Fele
Sociology and Social Research
University of Trento
Trento, Italy

ISBN 978-3-031-26238-8 ISBN 978-3-031-26239-5 (eBook)
https://doi.org/10.1007/978-3-031-26239-5

This Palgrave Macmillan imprint is published by the registered company Springer Nature Switzerland AG.
The registered company address is: Gewerbestrasse 11, 6330 Cham, Switzerland

Acknowledgements

The book is mainly based on previous publications (Fele, 2006, 2007, 2009, 2014, 2016), which have been considerably re-written for this occasion. In particular, I thank John Benjamins Publishing Company for granting the reprint of part of the publication "Requesting help with null or limited knowledge: Entitlements and responsibility in emergency calls", in *Communicating Certainty and Uncertainty in Medical, Supportive and Scientific Contexts*, edited by Andrzej Zuczkowski, Ramona Bongelli, Ilaria Riccioni and Carla Canestrari (2014) https://benjamins.com/catalog/ds.25.

My grateful thanks go to the director of CO 118 Trentino Emergenza, Alberto Zini, to Giorgio Folgheraiter and to all the emergency operators, for allowing me to enter their world and gain access to the data. All the doctors and all the operators at the emergency call and dispatch centre have been for me a lucid example of dedicated and careful professional work.

I am profoundly grateful to Sabine, who not only has helped me with German but also has been a great source of support. Her example has been a spur for me to do better. Her humour made the tiring days light. My heartfelt thanks go to her. When writing the book, I have always borne in mind what Luca and Marco would say when reading these pages. I hope that they will pass their severe scrutiny.

Adrian Belton has done outstanding work in proofreading the text. Alicia Chiodi helped me in editing the manuscript with attentive care.

References

Fele, G. (2006). La communication dans l'urgence. Les appels au secours téléphoniques. *Revue française de linguistique appliquée, 11*(2), 33–51.

Fele, G. (2007). La rinuncia all'agency: forme di cooperazione e di interazione sociale tra gli operatori dell'emergenza. In A. Donzelli & A. Fasulo (Eds.), *Agency e linguaggio: etnoteorie della soggettività e della responsabilità nell'azione sociale* (pp. 173–193). Meltemi.

Fele, G. (2009). Glosse e formulazioni. In L. Mariottini, M. E. Sciubba, & M. Fatigante (Eds.), *Lingua e società. Scritti in onore di Franca Orletti per il suo sessantesimo compleanno* (pp. 49–59). Franco Angeli.

Fele, G. (2014). Requesting help with null or limited knowledge. In A. Zuczkowski, R. Bongelli, I. Riccioni, & C. Canestrari (Eds.), *Communicating certainty and uncertainty in medical, supportive and scientific contexts* (pp. 139–156). John Benjamins.

Fele, G. (2016). Overcoming language barriers in emergency telephone calls. In A. F. Plastina (Ed.), *Challenging language barriers in the public service. An interdisciplinary perspective* (pp. 15–38). Aracne editrice.

Contents

List of Figures

List of Excerpts

CHAPTER 1

Introduction

Abstract This chapter is an introduction to the volume, where aims, methodology, context and analytical tenets are specified.

Keywords Conversation analysis • Emergency calls • Workplace studies • Transcription

Emergency situations are a particularly rich subject of study for researchers interested in social interaction and communication practices. It would seem that, in emergency situations, the normal procedures and routines that regulate matters in ordinary life are suddenly accelerated and assume an unexpected appearance. Emergency conditions concentrate collective relations, dynamics of meaning and communication processes to an extent not found in other social situations.

The interweaving of routine and urgency characterizes a certain number of professional activities in which, as the American sociologist E.C. Hughes (1971, p. 316) pointed out, "one man's routine of work is made up of the emergencies of other people". Thus, a large number of studies on the professional treatment of emergencies within organizational structures set up for this purpose have been conducted. In addition to ethnographies of the work that operators perform in the field—both in emergency vehicles (Hughes, 1980; Mannon, 1981; Metz, 1981; Palmer,

G. Fele, *Emergency Communication*,
https://doi.org/10.1007/978-3-031-26239-5_1

1983) and at the scene of an accident (Büscher, 2005)—important studies have focused on the work in emergency response centres as "coordination centres" (Martin et al., 2007; Suchman, 1993, 1996, 1997). The activities performed in these emergency response centres or Public Safety Answering Points (PSAP) that manage requests for help have been the subject of a growing number of studies in Europe, the United States, South America, South Africa and Japan.

One important direction of research on emergency response work has focused on communication between the citizen who calls with a request for help or assistance and the operator (a call-taker) who responds.[1] In accordance with the principles of conversation analysis (Sacks, 1992), this research analyses the social organization of emergency calls by following the sequential development of verbal interaction.[2] Studies on calls requesting an emergency response deal with the communicative process as a case of 'talk as work' (Drew & Heritage, 1992), or institutional interaction (Arminen, 2005). It is this aspect that is mainly dealt with in this book.

Conversation analysis (CA) or talk-in-interaction is an analytical approach that studies the organization of talk between 'parties' (Sacks et al., 1974).[3] A conversation is considered as a sequence of 'turns at talk'. There are methodical procedures to follow in taking turns (Sacks et al.,

[1] See Heritage and Clayman (2010), Drew and Walker (2010), Cromdal (2012), Garcia (2013), Gerwing (2015), Kevoe-Feldman (2019). The analysis of emergency calls was initiated and is inspired by the seminal work of Don Zimmerman (and colleagues). There is also a substantial amount of literature on helplines. For an early reference, see Baker et al. (eds.) 2005. For a review, see Bloch and Leydon (2019) and Hepburn et al. (2014). On childbirth helplines, see Kitzinger (2011), Potter and Hepburn (2003), and Hepburn (2005). On suicide helpline calls, see Iversen (2021). For a discussion of the difference between divergent ways of 'getting help' by telephone, and, in particular, for a comparison between helplines and emergency calls, see Francis and Hester (2004, chap. 6), and Kevoe-Feldman and Iversen (2022). For a comparison between emergency calls and other service calls, see Wakin and Zimmerman (1999). For telephone healthcare advice calls between nurses and callers, see Leydon et al. (2013); Leppänen (2010); Danby et al. (2009). For calls between call-takers employed by the emergency medical services call centre and callers from the general emergency call centre in the Western Cape (Cape Town, South Africa), see Rafaely and Whitehead (2020).

[2] Previous work on calls for help—mostly addressed to the police—is sparse (see Antunes & Scott, 1981; Bercal, 1970; Broadhead, 1986; Gilsinan, 1989; Shearing, 1974). For a symbolic interactionist perspective, see Manning (1988).

[3] There are several good introductory publications to conversation analysis. For a limited sample, see Heritage (1984); Maynard (2013); Sidnell (2013). See Clayman et al. (2022) and Lynch (2000) for an examination of the ethnomethodological roots of conversation analysis.

1974), just as there are in repairing troubles in talk (Hayashi et al., 2013; Schegloff et al., 1977). CA relies on the perspectives of participants in order to describe how 'parties' talk: that is to say, on adopting this approach, each participant is viewed as showing in each of his/her turns the 'interpretation' of what the other has just said in the previous turn; each next turn exhibits or embodies what a participant has understood of the previous turn. An emergency call is considered to be a particular case of talk-in-interaction. Compared to ordinary calls, those to emergency response centres exhibit a reduction and specialization of their organization: they are relatively brief communicative events, and they are focused on one main goal (Eglin & Wideman, 1986): that is, requesting, soliciting or asking for help and assistance. The work of the call-taker is to ascertain and examine step-by-step the caller's request, solicitation or demand before granting (or refusing) help. All this work must be done under strong time pressure, where the precision and accuracy of the reconstruction of the events at the basis of the emergency call collide with the necessity to act promptly. This book explores some of the situations where this tension between opposite requirements is clearest.

The last chapter of the book is inspired by the analytical principles of 'workplace studies' (Luff et al., 2000; Heath & Luff, 1996; Hindmarsh & Heath, 2007), and it is focused on how operators at emergency response centres (call-takers, dispatchers and supervisors) perform their tasks in a climate of intense collaboration (open or tacit) in which communication technology (radio, fixed and mobile telephones, fax machines, etc.) and information management (CAD, etc.) are part of a social and collaborative use of instruments. Workplace studies show that the resolution of ambiguities and the decision-making, the categorization and the classification of events are the product of subtle joint management by the operators working together on emergencies.

The book is based on analysis of audio and recorded real data, not on interviews or reconstructed scenarios. The recordings have been collected in different periods of fieldwork (which began in 2003 and is still ongoing) in three call and dispatch centres in Northern Italy. The main material on which the book is based derives from research conducted on the emergency call and dispatch centre Trentino Emergenza 118, a dedicated number to answer health and medical emergencies. At the time of writing, the organization of the emergency call and dispatch centres in Italy is undergoing legal and institutional change. A single Europe-wide emergency number (112) is being progressively adopted in several Regions, among them Trentino. This means that now there are two kinds of PSAP in place: one dedicated to answering all the calls made to the emergency number (first-level PSAP) and one mobilized according to three specific kinds of emergency (depending if one needs medical staff, police, or firefighters—second-level PSAP). My analysis is designed to raise analytical points and not to provide a description of different systems. I hope that its main findings will be of general interest, beyond national and organizational specificities—although, when relevant, I take those specificities into account.

The data were collected in 2003 for research that is still ongoing and amounted to about 45 hours of video recordings of ordinary working days, plus all the related incoming and outgoing audio communications via radio and telephone. The calls were transcribed and analysed according to the principles of conversation analysis (Hepburn & Bolden, 2013). Names and other identifying tokens were cancelled or altered for the sake of privacy.

The book is organized into seven chapters. In the second chapter, I focus on emergency calls in their overall structural organization. I describe their constituent parts, starting with the openings. I then consider the different ways in which help can be solicited by the caller. I examine the ways in which the call-taker assesses the credibility and the pertinence of the call. Thereafter, I analyse the ways in which the call can be brought to a close and the help granted. Finally, I examine difficulties that may arise in handling the call.

In the third chapter, I examine in particular the ways in which the place of the emergency may be formulated. How to locate the scene of an emergency is a major task for the call-takers. I examine different ways to describe places and the callers' orientation to the importance of locating the emergency. At the same time, part of the call-taker's job is to work the call so that the place of the emergency can be ascertained with precision. What emerges is that place descriptions are made not to describe a state of the world, but in order to be used, that is, made practically recognizable.

The fourth chapter deals with calls that are not emergency calls. In particular, I examine how callers design their turn so that the call-taker immediately realises that the call is not an emergency. I show that formulating the action one is doing is a powerful method to make clear what the speaker is doing. I analyse cases in which the caller uses a formulation to make it clear that she/he is asking for information, not asking for help.

The fifth chapter deals with a possible problem in calling for help. Often the call is made by a third person who has limited or no knowledge of what has generated the need for an emergency intervention. Claims by the caller of limited or no knowledge about the case are delicate interactional matters because the caller should be able to offer grounds for his/her request. I show the ways in which callers deal with this problematic aspect in their turns, and the conditions under which help is nevertheless granted even in the absence of information.

The sixth chapter deals with language difficulties in emergency calls due to the fact that the caller is not a speaker of the call-taker's language and that the call-taker does not understand the caller's language. Using a single case analysis, I focus on a call where a professional interpreter is sought. I describe the language trouble between caller and call-taker, the ways in which the professional interpreter was recruited, the conversation of the interpreter with the caller, and the interpreter's rendering of the caller's need. I argue that the work of the interpreter is less than that of a translation machine and more that of the coordinator of meanings and understandings.

The seventh chapter focuses on the tacit collaborative work between call-takers and dispatchers in dealing with emergency calls. I analyse the dispatch of aid as a collaborative product of dispatchers and call-takers alike through forms of complex interactional work. Besides considering the dispatch as a specific form of radio communication between the emergency call centre and the ambulance on the ground, I observe through the use of video recordings the subtle and delicate collaborative work of dispatchers and call-takers. This hidden work does not appear in any official records, but at the same time not only is it at the core of the activities in the emergency call centre, but it offers a splendid illustration of the subtle ways in which the organizational culture of emergency professionals reveals itself.

References

Antunes, G., & Scott, E. J. (1981). Calling the cops: Police telephone operators and citizen calls for service. *Journal of Criminal Justice, 9*, 165–179.

Arminen, I. (2005). *Institutional interaction: Studies of talk at work*. Ashgate.

Baker, C., Emmison, M., & Firth, A. (Eds.). (2005). *Calling for help: Language and social interaction in telephone helplines.* John Benjamins.

Bercal, T. E. (1970). Calls for police assistance: Consumer demands for governmental service. *American Behavioral Scientist, 13*, 681–691.

Bloch, S., & Leydon, G. (2019). Conversation analysis and telephone helplines for health and illness: A narrative review. *Research on Language and Social Interaction, 52*(3), 193–211.

Broadhead, R. S. (1986). Directing intervention from afar: The telephone dynamics of managing acute poisoning. *Journal of Health and Social Behavior, 27*, 303–319.

Büscher, M. (2005). Embodied conduct and movement in emergency teamwork. In L. Mondada (Ed.), *Gestures and the organisation of social interaction: Ethnomethodological and conversational perspectives.* Conference Proceedings. Lyon-France June 15–18. https://eprints.lancs.ac.uk/id/eprint/62088/1/Buscher_revised2706.pdf

Clayman, S. E., Heritage, J., & Maynard, D. W. (2022). The ethnomethodological lineage of conversation analysis. In D. W. Maynard & J. Heritage (Eds.), *The ethnomethodology program: Legacies and prospects* (pp. 252–286). Oxford University Press.

Cromdal, J. (2012). Conversation analysis and emergency calls. In C. Chapelle (Ed.), *The encyclopaedia of applied linguistics.* Wiley-Blackwell.

Danby, S., Butler, C. W., & Emmison, M. (2009). When "listeners can't talk": Comparing active listening in opening sequences of telephone and online counselling. *Australian Journal of Communication, 36*(3), 91–114.

Drew, P., & Heritage, J. (1992). Talk at work: An introduction. In P. Drew & J. Heritage (Eds.), *Talk at work: Interaction in institutional settings* (pp. 3–65). Cambridge University Press.

Drew, P., & Walker, T. (2010). Citizen's emergency calls to police: Requesting assistance in calls to the police. In M. Coulthard & A. Johnson (Eds.), *Handbook of forensic linguistic* (pp. 95–110). Routledge.

Eglin, P., & Wideman, D. (1986). Inequality in professional service encounters: Verbal strategies of control versus task performance in calls to the police. *Zeitschrift fur Soziologie, 15*(5), 341–362.

Francis, D., & Hester, S. (2004). *An invitation to ethnomethodology: Language, society and social interaction.* Sage.

Garcia, A. C. (2013). Routine service calls: Emergency calls to the police. In A. C. Garcia (Ed.), *An introduction to interaction: Understanding talk in formal and informal settings* (pp. 154–165). Bloomsbury.

Gerwing, J. (2015). Emergency telephone discourse. In K. Tracy, C. Ilie, & T. Sandel (Eds.), *The international encyclopedia of language and social interaction.* Wiley-Blackwell.

Gilsinan, J. F. (1989). They is clowning tough: 911 and the social construction of reality. *Criminology, 27*(2), 329–344.

Hayashi, M., Raymond, G., & Sidnell, J. (2013). Conversational repair and human understanding: An introduction. In M. Hayashi, G. Raymond, & J. Sidnell (Eds.), *Conversational repair and human understanding* (pp. 1–30). Cambridge University Press.

Heath, C., & Luff, P. (1996). Convergent activities: Line control and passenger information on the London underground. In Y. Engestrom & D. Middleton (Eds.), *Cognition and communication at work* (pp. 96–129). Cambridge University Press.

Hepburn, A. (2005). "You're not takin' me seriously": Ethics and asymmetry in calls to a child protection helpline. *Journal of Constructivist Psychology, 18*, 253–274.

Hepburn, A., & Bolden, G. B. (2013). The conversation analytic approach to transcription. In J. Sidnell & T. Stivers (Eds.), *The handbook of conversation analysis* (pp. 57–76). Wiley-Blackwell Publishing.

Hepburn, A., Wilkinson, S., & Butler, C. W. (2014). Intervening with conversation analysis in telephone helpline services: Strategies to improve effectiveness. *Research on Language and Social Interaction, 47*(3), 239–254.

Heritage, J. (1984). Conversation analysis. In J. Heritage (Ed.), *Garfinkel and ethnomethodology* (pp. 233–244). Polity Press.

Heritage, J., & Clayman, S. E. (2010). Calls for emergency service. In J. Heritage & S. Clayman (Eds.), *Talk in action: Interactions, identities, and institutions* (pp. 53–100). Wiley-Blackwell.

Hindmarsh, J., & Heath, C. (2007). Video-based studies of work practice. *Sociology Compass, 1*(1), 156–173.

Hughes, E. C. (1971). *The sociological eye*. Aldine Atherton.

Hughes, D. (1980). The ambulance journey as an information generating process. *Sociology of Health and Illness, 2*(2), 115–132.

Iversen, C. (2021). Making sense of experiences in suicide helpline calls: Offering empathy without endorsing suicidal ideation. *Sociology of Health & Illness, 43*(9), 2066–2084.

Kevoe-Feldman, H. (2019). Inside the emergency service call-center: Reviewing thirty years of language and social interaction research. *Research on Language and Social Interaction, 52*(3), 227–240.

Kevoe-Feldman, H., & Iversen, C. (2022). Approaching institutional boundaries: Comparative conversation analysis of practices for assisting suicidal callers in emergency and suicide helpline calls. *Journal of Pragmatics, 191*, 83–97.

Kitzinger, C. (2011). Working with childbirth helplines: The contributions and limitations of conversation analysis. In C. Antaki (Ed.), *Applied conversation analysis: Intervention and change in institutional talk* (pp. 98–118). Palgrave Macmillan.

Leppänen, V. (2010). Power in telephone advice nursing. *Nursing Inquiry, 17*(1), 15–26.

Leydon, G. M., Ekberg, K., & Drew, P. (2013). "How can I help?" Nurse call openings on a cancer helpline and implications for call progressivity. *Patient Education and Counseling, 92*(1), 23–30.

Luff, P., Hindmarsh, J., & Heath, C. (Eds.). (2000). *Workplace studies: Recovering work practice and informing system design*. Cambridge University Press.

Lynch, M. (2000). The ethnomethodological foundations of conversation analysis. *Text, 20*(4), 517–532.

Manning, P. F. (1988). *Symbolic communication. Signifying calls and the police response*. MIT Press.

Mannon, J. M. (1981). *Emergency encounters. A study of an ambulance service*. Kennikat Press.

Martin, D., O'Neill, J., Randall, D., & Rouncefield, M. (2007). How can I help you? Call centres, classification work and coordination. *Computer Supported Cooperative Work (CSCW), 16*(3), 231–264.

Maynard, D. W. (2013). Everyone and No one to turn to: Intellectual roots and contexts for conversation analysis. In J. Sidnell & T. Stivers (Eds.), *The handbook of conversation analysis* (pp. 11–31). Willey-Blackwell Publishing.

Metz, D. L. (1981). *Running hot. Structure and stress in ambulance work*. ABT Books.

Palmer, E. C. (1983). Trauma junkies and street work: Occupational behavior of paramedics and emergency medical technicians. *Urban Life, 12*(2), 162–183.

Potter, J., & Hepburn, A. (2003). "I'm a bit concerned": Early actions and psychological constructions in a child protection helpline. *Research on Language and Social Interaction, 36*(3), 197–240.

Rafaely, D., & Whitehead, K. A. (2020). Extraordinary emergencies: Reproducing moral discourses of the child in institutional interaction. *Pragmatics and Society, 11*(1), 45–69.

Sacks, H. (1992). *Lectures on conversation*. Blackwell.

Sacks, H., Schegloff, E. A., & Jefferson, G. (1974). A simplest systematics for the organization of turn-taking for conversation. *Language, 50*, 696–735.

Schegloff, E. A., Jefferson, G., & Sacks, H. (1977). The preference for self-correction in the organization of repair in conversation. *Language, 53*(2), 361–382.

Shearing, C. D. (1974). Dial-a-cop: A study of police mobilization. In R. L. Akers & E. Sagarin (Eds.), *Crime prevention and social control* (pp. 77–88). Praeger.

Sidnell, J. (2013). Basic conversation analytic methods. In J. Sidnell & T. Stivers (Eds.), *The handbook of conversation analysis* (pp. 77–99). Willey-Blackwell.

Suchman, L. (1993). Technologies of accountability: Of lizards and airplanes. In G. Button (Ed.), *Technology in working order: Studies of work, interaction and technology* (pp. 113–126). Routledge.

Suchman, L. (1996). Constituting shared workspaces. In Y. Engestroem & D. Middleton (Eds.), *Cognition and communication at work* (pp. 35–60). Cambridge University Press.
Suchman, L. (1997). Centers of coordination. A case and some themes. In L. Resnick, R. Säljö, C. Pontecorvo, & B. Burge (Eds.), *Discourse, tools and reasoning. Essays on situated cognition* (pp. 41–62). Springer.
Wakin, M. A., & Zimmerman, D. H. (1999). Reduction and specialization in emergency and directory assistance calls. *Research on Language and Social Interaction, 32*(4), 409–437.

CHAPTER 2

The Organization of Emergency Calls

Abstract In this chapter, I analyse the organization of emergency calls. I describe the overall structural organization (Robinson, Overall structural organization. In J. Sidnell & T. Stivers (Eds.), *The handbook of conversation analysis* (pp. 257–280). Wiley-Blackwell, 2012) and its constituent parts. The openings of emergency calls are particularly interesting to analyse because it is there that the status of a call as relative to an event requiring help (or not) is made evident. I consider the different ways in which help can be solicited. I then examine the ways in which the call-taker assesses the credibility and the pertinence of the call, doing so by means of a series of questions. Thereafter, I analyse the ways in which the call can be brought to a close and the help granted. Finally, I examine difficulties that may arise in handling the call.

Keywords Call openings • Requests for assistance • Description of problems • Interrogative series • Call closings • Troubles with the caller

1 Structural Organization

A call to an emergency number is a highly specialized form of talk oriented to a specific goal, and can be described as a typical, recursive sequence of elements (Drew & Heritage, 1992, pp. 43–45). According to Zimmerman (1984, 1992a, p. 419; 1992b, p. 37), in each call one observes the

G. Fele, *Emergency Communication*,
https://doi.org/10.1007/978-3-031-26239-5_2

presence of five main phases: (1) opening and identification; (2) the request for assistance; (3) a series of questions on the part of the operator, who tries to obtain the information necessary for the intervention; (4) his/her response to the request for help; (5) the closing.

These phases are shown in the following excerpt, which is the transcript of a call to the Italian medical emergency number 118[1] following the runway overrun of an aircraft on the morning of 30 July 1997 at the Peretola Airport of Florence, Italy[2]:

Excerpt 2.1 Florence Airport[3]

```
-----------------------------------------------------------------
              ((tone))
01 Ctaker     centodiciotto Firenze.                            1
              one one eight Florence
02 Caller     centodiciotto,
              one one eight,
-----------------------------------------------------------------
03            quattro ambulanze immediatamente in aeroporto,
              four ambulances immediately to the airport        2
04            anzi no quattro, più che potete.
              actually, not four, as many as you can.
05            c'è stato un incidente.
              there has been an accident.
-----------------------------------------------------------------
06 Ctaker     signora, dove?
              madam, where?
07 Caller     in aeroporto, a Firenze Peretola.
              at the airport, Firenze Peretola.
08 Ctaker     <aeroporto> ((while writing))
              <airport>
```

(continued)

[1] For a comparison between Italian and English in emergency calls, see Monzoni and Zorzi (2003).

[2] Details about the incident can be found here: https://aviation-safety.net/database/record.php?id=19970730-0 (last access 9/8/2022).

[3] The audio file was available at N&A September 1997, page 3.

Excerpt 2.1 (continued)

09	Caller	ma immediatamente!	
		but immediately	
10	Ctaker	<Peretola> ((while writing))	
		<Peretola>	**3**
11	Caller	è la direzione dell'aeroporto.	
		it's the airport control centre.	
12	Ctaker	che tipo di incidente è.	
		what kind of accident is it.	
13	Caller	eh, un aereo è andato fuori pista. veloci!	
		eh, an airplane has skidded off the runway. quick!	
14	Ctaker	bene. si manda subito qualcuno.	**4**
		okay. we'll send someone immediately.	
15	Caller	grazie. ((click))	**5**
		thanks.	

We find in this extract the five characteristic phases of this type of call: the opening and identification (lines 1–2); the request for help (lines 3–4); a series of questions by the operator (lines 5–12); the response to the request for help (line 13); the closing (line 14). The opening of the conversation is accomplished in the first phase. The opening of the call is designed by the call-taker to orient the caller towards the institutional task of emergency numbers. Zimmerman (1992b) and Wakin and Zimmerman (1999) show that, in emergency calls, the trajectory of the call is significantly different from that of ordinary non-service calls: in particular, they find that calls to emergency numbers erase, anticipate or reposition some of the 'canonical' components of the opening sequence of ordinary calls. The organization of emergency calls is aimed specifically at gathering information relevant to the event and processing it with minimal delay. Zimmerman (1992b) and Wakin and Zimmerman (1999) analyse the way in which call-takers are oriented first to the task of understanding what has happened and then of transmitting the relevant information to the dispatchers who are going to send help on the ground. This phase of dispatching will be analysed in the sixth chapter. The focus in what follows is on the five phases of the emergency call in more detail.

2 The Components of the Opening of Emergency Calls and the Request for Assistance

I analyse the first exchange, the call-taker's first turn, and the caller's first turn. I begin with a comparison between ordinary calls and calls to an emergency number.

2.1 *The Opening*

The opening of any telephone conversation constitutes a 'dense' interactional space (Schegloff, 1968, 2002a) where a series of tasks must be completed in order to proceed ahead in the conversation. The participants must position themselves reciprocally and precisely in a few turns of talk and a few fleeting moments. Callers and recipients do not have the visual resources that make it possible to recognize the other speaker through visual access. In telephone calls, whatever the business is, it is done by means of the voice, spoken words and auditory cues. Consequently, as Svensson and Hällgren (2018) state, also emergency call-takers make sense of calls in what can be defined "a sensory deprived setting".[4]

Ordinary call openings are constructed using elementary resources: relatively simple, few and recurrent lexical items that constitute brief, compact turns of talk. There are no sophisticated phrases or syntactic constructions. Schegloff (1986) has identified in the opening phase of ordinary telephone conversations an organization composed of at least three (or four) types of sequences that can be completed before the first topic is introduced. See the following excerpt (Schegloff, 1986, p. 115; transcription simplified):

[4] Neustaedter et al. (2017, 2019) and Landgren and Bergstrand (2010) show the potential of video calling services for the management of emergencies.

Excerpt 2.2 From Schegloff, 1986, p. 123

```
 0 ring
 1 R Hello::,
 2 C H'llo, Clara?
 3 R Yeh,
 4 C Hi. Bernie.
 5 R Hi Bernie.
 6 C How're you.
 7 R I'm alright,
     How're you.
 8 C Okay:?
 9 R Good.
10 C Laura there?
```

The first sequence consists of a 'summons-answer pair' (lines 0–1); the second sequence is designed to identify the caller and receiver (lines 2–4); the third sequence is that of greetings (lines 4–5); the fourth sequence is constituted by a sequence of exchanges of pleasantries and niceties (lines 6–9). It is after the end of the last exchange of pleasantries that the first opportunity to introduce the reason for the call arises (as in line 10): in general, at this point the interaction has unfolded in such a way that the caller is well placed to introduce the reason for the call. In ordinary calls, the interaction proceeds with a step-by-step sequential procedure (Schegloff, 1986). It is interesting to note that before the caller can properly begin to talk about something, the caller and the receiver secure the communication channel and align their mutual identities (Schegloff, 1979). The opening phase plays a fundamental role in what has been called the 'positioning problem' (Schegloff, 1986, pp. 116–117) in ordinary telephone conversations. The positioning problem consists in the fact that the reason for the call is formulated 'in a certain place', and has to be positioned at a certain point in the conversation. The initial procedures of ordinary calls make it possible to set up a first structural place that can accommodate the reason for the call, just after the completion of these initial procedures.

The organization of the call opening that I have summarized has been described as standard in American English landline phone calls, even if Schegloff (2002b) conducted a comparative discussion on the cultural variations of telephone openings. There have also been studies on openings in mobile phone calls. Arminen and Leinonen (2006, p. 362), on studying Finnish mobile phone conversations, found that mobile calls differ systematically from landline call openings. As they write, "The major difference is that the answers to the summons of a mobile call treat the summons as being personalized in giving information on the caller, and allowing the answer to be designed accordingly." We may say that, in these cases, the sequence is shorter than that of the landline calls.

In any case, what happens in the opening sequence of emergency calls is very different from the patterns just described.[5] The sequence is much shorter and more specialized (Whalen & Zimmerman, 1987; Wakin & Zimmerman, 1999). Let us return to Excerpt 2.1:

Excerpt 2.3 Florence Airport, Lines 01, 02, Section 1—From Excerpt 2.1

```
01 Ctaker    centodiciotto Firenze.
             one one eight Florence.
02 Caller    centodiciotto,
             one one eight,
```

We can see that the call begins with a categorical identification of the service requested (line 1: "one one eight Firenze"). Just as when one is dealing with a policeman, a military officer, a doctor or someone wearing a uniform or a coat (Fussell, 2002), the receiver immediately discloses the type of identity relevant to the interaction in the call. Similarly, in an emergency call, the person who answers the phone immediately defines the type of service that caller has reached.

The response to the summons has been modulated according to national and organizational constraints in two main ways, and also a combination of the two, mainly by stating the number that the caller has

[5] See in particular Zimmerman (1992a). For a discussion of the different ways of opening emergency calls and their interactional consequences, see Cromdal et al. (2012, 2012); Koole and Verberg (2017); Penn et al. (2017); Vaajala et al. (2013). See also Danby et al. (2005) for openings in calls to a kid helpline, and Leydon et al. (2013) on openings of a cancer helpline; Vinkhuyzen et al. (2006) on openings of calls to a financial services organization; González-Martínez (2017) on openings of calls between nurses and porters at a hospital in Switzerland.

reached—like 118, 115 or 113 in Italy, 112 as the single emergency number in Europe, 911 in the United States, 999 in the United Kingdom, 119 in Japan, and so on—or by explicitly naming the service provided, like "emergency", "police", and so on, alerting the caller as to the kind of the service that she/he has reached (Cromdal et al., 2012). The definition of categorical identity in emergency calls not only has the same function as the "hello" with which ordinary calls are answered—that is, answering the summons—but it also has fundamental consequences for the ensuing activity.[6] The categorical identity makes it perceptually hearable to the caller that a channel is open and that the (institutional) identity of the receiver is established. In emergency calls, this makes it clear to the caller that his/her first turn is entirely concerned with the reason for the call. In my data, the caller's first turn does not usually present any personal identification on his/her part,[7] and no greeting is offered[8] The first caller's turn is instead entirely occupied with the presentation of the problem and the request for help. The identities relevant to the encounter are established in just two rounds of talk. Verbal exchanges entail that there is a speaker and a listener (and that these roles are interchangeable); in a telephone conversation, the rights and duties of the caller and respondent are established. In a call to an emergency number, the participants work within the contingencies of the call to align themselves reciprocally as "benefactors and beneficiaries" (Clayman & Heritage, 2014); "Nutznießer" and "Wohltäter" (Bergmann, 1992[9]); "citizen complainant" and "call-taker" (Zimmerman, 1998); "service seeker" and "service provider" (Raymond & Zimmerman, 2007, 2016), "help seeker" and "help provider" (Cromdal et al., 2012, p. 373)[10]; in other words, one participant—the caller—as a "citizen" or "person in need of help", and the other—the call-taker—as "the one who undertakes the necessary steps to ensure that the help

[6] See Garcia (2022) to learn how call-takers use racial/ethnic categories to describe persons of interest such as suspects, victims or persons needing assistance.

[7] But see, for example, Vaajala et al. (2013), where it seems that Finnish emergency calls have personal names as a regular feature of their openings. When personal names do not appear as a regular feature of the openings, it is interesting to observe what kind of interactional work personal names do in the call when they appear. See Chap. 3.

[8] See how greetings and self-identification are instead present in calls to a (Uruguayan) carer service by relative or next of kin (of the patient) to request a day/night carer for the patient who is in hospital (Reiter, 2006).

[9] Quoted by Koole and van Burgsteden (2022, p. 273).

[10] To be noted here is that the caller often calls on behalf of a third party: the caller is often not himself a "victim" or a "patient". For an analysis of calls to a victim support helpline seeking help for others, see Tennent (2021).

required is provided". The task of defining institutional identities, accomplished in just two turns of speaking, sets the expectations for the rest of the interaction. The response of emergency operators is not intended to allow for voice recognition, as is the case with ordinary calls, but instead to provide an institutional identity that the service itself requires and that the caller expects. Indeed, as Zimmerman (1992b, p. 43) points out, "in dialing the advertised number of the police or fire department, callers expect to connect with an answerer acting in the capacity of an agent of that organization, an identity that the answerer's self-identification confirms". It is in this sense that the response of the emergency operator exhibits the characteristic of being specialized for a particular purpose within the interaction in progress (Wakin & Zimmerman, 1999; Whalen & Zimmerman, 1987). Thus, Wilson (1991, p. 34) observes that "at this point, the relation between the parties has been established in terms of the manifest business of the agency the caller has intentionally reached, namely the dispatching of help in response to requests or reports of trouble. [...] In sum, caller and answerer have established the potential relevance of a mutual categorization of each other as citizen complainant and complaint taker, where these categorical identities are specifically tied to the particular organization the caller has reached".[11]

2.2 *The Request for Assistance*[12]

Let us now consider how the emergency call proceeds. After the operator's turn to answer the call (the ringing of the phone), the caller has the right to talk for the first time. We have seen that, in my data, the caller does not identify himself/herself. In calls for help, the emergency nature of the call is indexed by the fact that the caller usually moves immediately to the formulation of the problem, at the first opportunity at his/her disposal.[13]

[11] In this way, also silent calls can be treated as implying a request for help. See Kevoe-Feldman and Sutherland (2018) for an analysis of the treatment of silent calls by call-takers.

[12] On requesting in talk-in-interaction, see Drew and Couper-Kuhlen (2014).

[13] When the call-taker follows the dispatch protocol called Medical Priority Dispatch System (MPDS), the first question is intended to obtain information regarding the location of the accident ("*ambulance what's the exact address of the emergency*"), not the reason for the call. In these cases, the caller's first turn can pre-empt the reason of the call. See Riou et al. (2018) for how call-takers manage this pre-emption.

Excerpt 2.4 Florence Airport, Lines 03, 04, 05, Section 1—From Excerpt 2.1

```
03 Caller   quattro ambulanze immediatamente in aeroporto,
            four ambulances immediately to the airport
04          anzi no quattro, più che potete.
            actually, not four, as many as you can.
05          c'è stato un incidente.
            there has been an accident.
```

This is the case of lines 3–4 of Excerpt 2.1: "four ambulances immediately to the airport. Actually, not four, as many as you can. There has been an accident". We can see that in this extended turn of the caller there is a request for a here-and-now intervention. It is a strong example of a request for immediate action couched in the imperative (Sorjonen et al., 2017). Here the immediacy and urgency of the action requested are left grammatically incomplete, with the minimal linguistic form of the verb unspoken (what is missing is something like "send!"). The imperative form of the requested assistance conveys the meaning that the "actions need to be done immediately, with serious consequences in case of their delay" (Sorjonen et al., 2017, p. 13). No mitigation towards the commitment of the emergency service is to be found in the design of the turn; instead, the urgency of the requested assistance is heightened by the request to send "as many ambulances as you can". This turn is designed to maximize the urgency and ground the request urging the call-taker to act immediately.[14] It makes the call-taker immediately responsible for taking the necessary steps to deploy assistance.[15]

[14] Larsen (2013, p. 228) shows that "when the callers choose a request format that makes a strong claim of entitlement, then the call takers also treat them as entitled by engaging in dispatch-relevant questioning without asking for any information about the incident. Conversely, when the callers choose a request format that only makes a weak claim of entitlement, then the call takers treat them as not necessarily entitled to have their requests granted".

[15] "The use of an imperative turn format often displays that the action nominated is compatible with the recipient's on-going course of action and/or promotes an activity that the recipient is committed to. In doing so, it implies an assumption that the action nominated is necessary and self-evidently grantable from the participants' shared perspective" (Sorjonen et al., 2017, p. 14). See also Craven and Potter (2010).

Not always does the caller's first turn in emergency calls show this pattern: rather, it seems that callers often limit their turn to presenting the case to the call-taker.[16]

Let us consider this next excerpt, which, like the previous one, deals with an aircraft accident[17]:

Excerpt 2.5 Verona Airport[18]

01 Ctaker	sì, Verona emergenza?
	yes, Verona emergency?
02 Caller	eh, hem, in località, Poiane, in via Dossobuono,
	eh, ehm, in the Poiane countryside, Dossobuono Road
03	a Sommacampagna, è appena caduto un aereo.
	Sommacampagna, a plane has just crashed.
04 Ctaker	un aereo?
	a plane?

In this call, we do not see a proper 'request' for assistance in the caller's first turn, which is entirely occupied by a report of an accident, a description of an event, a formulation of a problem,[19] while there is no fully explicit request for assistance (Whalen & Zimmerman, 1987, 1990; Zimmerman, 1984).[20] It seems that the situation described deserved in itself the maximum attention of the call-taker, and that it was considered enough to prompt the rapid dispatch of assistance. In the excerpt, we see a confirmation check issued by the call-taker (line 4) with which confirmation of part of the initial description of a rather unexpected event can be secured from the caller.

[16] "In a study conducted for the (London) Metropolitan Police Service, in the majority (a little under 80%) of calls callers only reported an incident without overtly requesting police assistance" (Drew & Walker, 2010, p. 97).

[17] Details about the incident can be found here: https://aviation-safety.net/database/record.php?id=19951213-0 (last access 9/8/2022).

[18] The audio file was available at N&A, last update: 10 January 1996.

[19] On the different caller strategies and the responses of the call-taker, see Imbens-Bailey and McCabe (2000).

[20] See also Fox and Heinemann (2021) on the role of declarative sentences of trouble in service encounters.

Imperatives-directives and descriptions can be considered two ways in which the assistance of the emergency system can be mobilized (Stivers & Rossano, 2010; Taleghani-Nikazm et al., 2020) by the caller. Zimmerman (1992a, pp. 435–411) identifies other ways to present the reason for the call, mainly with the use of explicit forms of request. See the following excerpts:

Excerpt 2.6 An Ambulance Is Needed

```
01 Ctaker   centodiciotto
            one one eight
02 Caller   eh sì buonasera senta servirebbe penso un'ambulanza
            eh yes good evening I think an ambulance is needed
03          all'altezza dell'Hotel Torbine
            up near Hotel Torbine
04          è stato- un bambino con una bicicletta,
            there was- a kid on a bike,
05          è stato credo urtato, si è fatto male,
            he has been knocked down, I think, he's been hurt,
06          adesso sta a terra
            now he's lying on the ground
```

Excerpt 2.7 Can You Send an Ambulance?

```
05 Ctaker   centodiciotto?
            one one eight
06 Caller   buon giorno, senta, può mandare un'autoambulanza m::
            good morning, listen, can you send an ambulance m::
            e[: in corso Torrini
            e:: to Torrini Avenue
07 Ctaker    [dove?
             where?
```

In Excerpt 2.6, the request from the caller is expressed in terms of need, even in an impersonal and conditional form (line 2: "I think an ambulance is needed"): the request for help imposes constraints on the call-taker to fulfil the request, even if the beneficiary of the help requested is not the caller. Moreover, the caller qualifies his request with a personal assessment of the situation ("I think"), thereby expressing not professional expertise but only his lay individual impression.

In Excerpt 2.7 (line 6: "can you send an ambulance"), the request is cast in terms of the possibility or impossibility for the receiver to comply with the request. As Deppermann and Gubina (2021) write, "It has been shown that *Can you X*?-requests are used if granting is potentially problematic due to (1) the recipient's involvement in a different course of action, which must be abandoned when complying [...]; (2) the requester's low entitlement to request the action; (3) recipient's previously displayed resistance to comply; and (4) a high degree of imposition on the recipient" (Deppermann & Gubina, 2021, pp. 186–187). Especially significant for requests to an emergency number are the terms indexed by Deppermann and Gubina as (1), (2) and (4): when the caller casts his/her request for help in a "can you" format, he/she shows awareness that the call may be an intrusion in the activities of the emergency service; that the call may concern matters less urgent than those which the emergency service is dealing with at the moment; that the deployment of help may divert resources from other emergency sites; and that the caller is not in a position to be the final judge of the seriousness of the ongoing situation.

In sum, when making a request, the caller shows that he is oriented to the contingencies associated with fulfilling the requested action and to the recipient's ability or willingness to carry out the requested action (Curl & Drew, 2008). At the same time, in the way that the request turn is formulated, the caller shows his/her entitlement to have the request granted: as Drew and Walker (2010, p. 100) observe, "these forms, ranging from imperatives through to conditional forms with 'I wonder if...' prefaces, lie along a cline from those which encode high entitlement and low contingency, to those which encode the reverse, that is high contingency and low entitlement."

3 The Interrogative Series

We have seen that requesting help and assistance is not a matter per se of securing the deployment of resources in order to cope with the emergency described. As Heritage and Clayman (2010) efficaciously put it, "calling 911 is not like ordering a pizza" (p. 69) (see also Whalen et al., 1988, p. 346)[21]: the service requested from an emergency call centre has to be carefully screened and verified by the call-taker and justified and substantiated by evidence and authenticity by the caller.[22] Whalen and Zimmerman (1987) (see also Zimmerman, 1998, pp. 101–105) speak of an "interrogative series": that is, a series of questions oriented to the genuineness of the problem and its importance (Heritage & Clayman, 2010).[23] Help requests that contain no information about the nature of the problem, thus soliciting a response without providing the reason for the request, are not sufficient to activate the deployment of help. Satisfaction of the request is therefore not immediate: the operators actively seek a certain amount of information before they can actually satisfy the request.

Let us go back to the first excerpt.

[21] Interestingly, 'ordering a pizza' from an emergency number may be an urgent plea for help by women in dangerous situations like domestic violence. On the call-taker's work to diagnose a pizza order as a request for help, see Albert et al. (2019). On women's disclosures of violence in calls for help to a victim support agency, see Tennent and Weatherall (2019).

[22] See also Emmison and Danby (2007). Kent and Antaki (2020) show that the call-taker's first substantive question already carries a diagnosis of the merits of the caller's case, projecting acceptance or refusal. Riou et al. (2017) studied the impact of linguistic variation in the delivery of the prompt "okay, tell me exactly what happened" by the call-taker on the response by the caller.

[23] Emergency call and dispatch centres have to deal also with a certain amount of hoax calls. See Weatherall et al. (2016) for a treatment of prank calls in an Australian children's counselling helpline calls.

Excerpt 2.8 Florence Airport, Lines from 06 to 13, Section 3—From Excerpt 2.1

06	Ctaker	signora, dove?
		madam, where?
07	Caller	in aeroporto, a Firenze Peretola.
		at the airport, Firenze Peretola.
08	Ctaker	<aeroporto> *((scrivendo))*
		<airport> ((while writing))
09	Caller	ma immediatamente!
		but immediately
10	Ctaker	<Peretola> *((scrivendo))*
		<Peretola> ((while writing))
11	Caller	è la direzione dell'aeroporto.
		it's the airport control centre.
12	Ctaker	che tipo di incidente è.
		what kind of accident is it.
13	Caller	eh, un aereo è andato fuori pista. veloci!
		eh, an airplane has skidded off the runway. quick!

In the excerpt, line 6, the call-taker checks again the site of the emergency (even if the caller had already packaged her first turn with a formulation of the place), engendering a reformulation of the place by the caller, who further specifies the location of the accident (not just "at the airport", but at the "airport Firenze Peretola", the international airport of Florence). In line 12, the call-taker asks for information regarding the kind of accident. Where the accident has happened[24] and what has happened are the basic items of information that are sought by the call-taker before granting the request for intervention (Mellinger, 1992).

Not having a reliable description of what has happened strongly impinges on the delivery of help. See the following excerpt:

[24] On the inquiry about the place, see Chap. 2.

Excerpt 2.9 The Machine Shop

```
01 Ctaker   centodiciotto?
            one one eight?
02 Caller   centodiciotto, qua la officina meccanica di Vigarona
            one one eight, the machine shop of Vigarona here
03 Ctaker   sì, cosa è succes[so?
            yes, what has happened?
04 Caller                    [serve urgentemente un ambulanza,
                              an ambulance is needed urgently,
05          si è fatto male un ragazzo.
            a guy has got hurt.
06 Ctaker   mi dica cosa gli è successo.
            tell me what has happened to him.
07 Caller   beh, non, non le so dire.
            well, I don't-, I don't know what to tell you.
08          è in terra svenuto.
            he's lying on the ground unconscious.
09 Ctaker   è per terra svenuto.
            he's lying on the ground unconscious.
10          lo vede respirare?
            do you see him breathing?
11 Caller   eh, adesso "lo vede",
            well, now "do you see him",
12          le ho telefonato per [(     )
            I called you for (     )
13 Ctaker                         [ma non "si è fatto male",
                                   but not "he's got hurt",
14          signore, bisogna che mi dica bene=
            sir, what is needed is that you tell me clearly=
15          =cosa è successo,
            =what has happened.
16          perché se c'è bisogno mando anche l'elicottero.
            because if it is needed I'll even send the helicopter.
17 Caller   eh, aspetti un attimo.
            eh, wait a moment.
        ((call continues))
```

We can see in this excerpt that the caller self-identifies not with his name but with his organizational connection (line 2: "the machine shop of Vigarona here"), where a categorical self-identification (Zimmerman, 1992a) provides both some warrant regarding the reported case and an identification of the location of the accident.[25] After the call-taker has started the interrogative series regarding the reason for the call (line 3: "what has happened?"), the caller solicits an ambulance with a turn designed as a high entitlement and low contingency request (line 4: "an ambulance is needed urgently") and a description, a declarative sentence informing[26] the call-taker about some trouble (line 5: "a guy has got hurt") but providing no details regarding the case, using a generic reference term (Tracy & Anderson, 1999, pp. 207–210) to identify the victim. The description is treated by the call-taker as insufficient to justify the immediate dispatch of help. The call-taker therefore continues the interrogative series with a question intended to obtain more details about the case and possibly also the dynamics of the accident and not just its results (line 6: "tell me what has happened to him"). The call-taker's turn projects an extended caller's turn—a narrative—in response. From this moment on, interactional problems start to appear. First, the caller fails to provide more details about the development of the event, but only its results (lines 7–8: "I don't know what to tell you. he's lying on the ground unconscious").[27] Then, after the call-taker makes a specific enquiry (line 9: "do you see him breathing?",)[28] the caller shows that he does not have first-hand knowledge of the event and that the person who needs assistance

[25] To be noted is that in Excerpt 2.1 the caller identifies herself in the call with a categorical self-identification ("a communication from 'my organization' to 'your organization', that is, as a report of a 'responsible party'", Zimmerman, 1998, p. 100). But she does so only later in the call (line 11: "it's the airport control centre") as a way to hasten the mobilization of help as a consequence of the previous management of the request by the call-taker (considered too slow) and to ground her request as coming from the most authoritative and reliable source available on the scene, not just from a private citizen (as the call-taker took the caller to be—see line 5: "madam, where?").

[26] On "informings" as recruitment in nurses' intrahospital telephone calls, see González-Martínez and Drew (2021).

[27] More on callers' "I don't knows" in Chap. 4.

[28] Berdowski et al. (2009), in quantitative analysis of the interaction between callers and call-takers, analyse how and when the question on "breathing" was actually made by call-takers, as a potential trigger for discovering a cardiac arrest. See also Riou et al. (2018).

is not in his field of vision (line 10: "now 'do you see him'", meaning something like, "do not ask now if I see him; this is a question impossible for me to answer"). The call-taker's question is taken by the caller to be a complaint about his limited knowledge. The caller expresses a rebuttal implying that he has no responsibility (Monzoni, 2009a, 2009b) for his limited knowledge, and he begins to show signs of procedural impatience (line 11: "I called you for ((incomprehensible))"), protesting about the delay with which his initial urgent request is being processed. The call-taker interrupts his protests by explicitly referring to his initial unsatisfactory formulation of the problem and then asks him for a more precise description of the event.

Between the call-taker and the caller, there is no longer that natural reciprocal alignment which favours the progressivity of an emergency call (Vaajala et al., 2013; Perera et al., 2020). In this case, the caller walks away from the phone—presumably in order to verify the facts—while the call-taker, via radio, dispatches an ambulance to the machine shop (not indicated in the transcript). The first problem, therefore, is that the caller had no direct access to the case, and was not a witness to the incident that was at the origin of the call. As we have seen, the caller gradually discovers how the organization works: a simple request for help does not result in the expected response unless a reasonable and reliable rationale for it is provided (Whalen & Zimmerman, 1990; Heritage & Clayman, 2010).[29]

Other calls begin with an account of the event that is less concise than a simple announcement. 'Reports' usually consist of declarative statements that inform the call-taker about the problem and concisely state the problem for which intervention is requested. However, callers have also been conceded the opportunity to tell a story, a narrative, that leads to identification of the problem, thus providing some additional contextual elements. In this way, the caller has an opportunity to fully describe not only the incident but also how she/he has come to know about the event and his/her relation with it. See the following excerpt:

[29] For an analysis of an ill-fated case where the call-taker came to doubt a caller who was reporting a genuine emergency, see Garcia and Parmer (1999). See also Garcia (2015) for an analysis of another tragic real case in which the caller failed to convince the call-taker that the request for service was urgent.

Excerpt 2.10 A Man Who Is Lying in a Flowerbed

```
01 Ctaker    centodiciotto
             one one eight
02 Caller    pronto buongiorno
             hello good morning
03 Ctaker    buongiorno
             good morning
04 caller    sono [nome] [cognome] di Relago, sono qua a Torgo
             I am [name] [surname] from Relago, I am here in Torgo
05 Ctaker    sì
             yes
06 Caller    davanti al bar al Toletta, ce n'è uno,
             in front of Bar Toletta, there is a person,
07           c'è un signore che è sdraiato qui sull'aiola
             there is a man who is lying here in the flowerbed
08           [che non sta bene=
             who is not well=
09 Ctaker    [sì
              yes
10 Caller    =penso io, non lo so, no?, io,
             =I think, I don't know, right?, I,
11           è qui sdraiato sull'aiola,
             he's lying in the flowerbed
12 Ctaker    [sì
              yes
13 Caller    [però non vorrei che andasse via mentre io son qua,
              but I wouldn't want him to go away while I am here,
14           perché adesso si sta movendo vedo
             because now I see he is moving
```

It is interesting how the caller uses his first turn at talk: in these first introductory lines, the call resembles a telephone call between unacquainted persons. The caller does not take the opportunity to immediately state the reason for the call; instead, he acknowledges having reached the number ("hello"), greets the respondent ("good morning") and identifies himself with his personal and family name,[30] before saying from where he is calling (lines 2, 4)—all these are considered by the call-taker as the preliminary elements of a story to come, and he gives a signal that the caller can continue (line 5: "yes"). The caller then describes a state of affairs from his personal perspective as a first-hand witness (lines 6–8: "in front of Bar Toletta, there is a person, there is a man who is lying here in the flowerbed who is not well"). In this extended turn, there is no explicit request for intervention: the description of the problem is characterized by low entitlement and high contingency, given that the caller gives only his lay opinion, not one based on professional expertise (lines 8, 10: "who is not well, I think, I don't know, right?"). His evaluation is based only on 'a strange fact' (line 11: "he's lying in the flowerbed") and no other details are given to the call-taker regarding the reason for his evaluation that the man is not feeling well. The caller says how he has come to know about the problem and that he is near a person with whom, however, he has no links (the person supposedly needing help is described as "a man"). The fact that the caller is a first-hand witness is shown also by the fact that he describes what he is seeing ("now I see he is moving"). That the victim seems to be moving is the reason for the concern that the caller expresses to the call-taker.

Zimmerman (1992a, p. 439) has observed that often in callers' reports there are details "within which both the features of the event and the grounds for claiming knowledge of them (the practical epistemology of their discovery) are provided" (see also Whalen & Zimmerman, 1990). Zimmerman (ibid.) adds: "The narrative format appears to furnish callers with the resources to pursue the mobilization of response to a possibly ambiguous problem, and to package their report in a way that exhibits their status as ordinary, disinterested, reasonable witnesses" (see also Bergmann, 1992). Differently from what occurs in announcements (with or without a direct request)—where events are presented in such a way that the reasonableness of the emergency call is immediately apparent—in the case of narratives callers often present events that are not immediately recognizable as emergencies requiring definite and immediate action by an organization (Sharrock & Turner, 1978, p. 179; cf. also Whalen et al., 1988, p. 346; Tracy & Agne, 2002 on family disputes). In these cases, call-takers invite the production of stories so that the callers can furnish better descriptions of the event and the basis of the (caller's) assessment of it as an emergency. And in any case, the final assessment of whether the case requires action is made by the call-takers (Meehan, 1989).[31] Whether a caller engages in an announcement, an account or a story has

[30] Interesting is the presence of the personal and family name here, in an environment where usually there is no other way to make the call authentic and worthy of acceptance.

[31] Callers not been interrogated accurately enough is a source of errors and underestimation of the situation (Palma et al., 2014).

consequences for the nature and extent of the questions that follow and consequently for the more or less rapid granting of the requested help.

4 Granting the Request and Thanking

We have seen that an emergency call is based on a request for assistance issued by the caller. Granting the assistance is not an immediate response; instead, the request is subjected to the scrutiny of the call-taker who needs to ascertain its genuineness and importance (Heritage & Clayman, 2010). When the case is sufficiently clear for all practical purposes, the call-taker's decision is communicated to the caller. It is as if the first part of an adjacency pair (the request), separated from the second part (the response) by an inserted sequence of questions and answers, is finally granted (Wilson, 1991). Let us return to the first call:

Excerpt 2.11 Granting the Request, Lines from 01 to 05, 14, 15—From Excerpt 2.1

```
01 Ctaker    centodiciotto Firenze.
             one one eight Florence
02 Caller    centodiciotto,
             one one eight,
03           quattro ambulanze immediatamente in aeroporto, REQUEST->-┐
             four ambulances immediately at the airport               |
04           anzi no quattro, più che potete.                         |
             actually not four, as many as you can.                   |
05           c'è stato un incidente.                                  |
             there has been an accident.                              |
                                                                      |
             ...(8 lines omitted) INTERROGATION SERIES                |
                                                                      |
14 Ctaker    bene. si manda subito qualcuno. GRANTING the REQUEST <---┘
             okay. we'll send someone immediately.
15 Caller    grazie. ((click))
             thanks.
```

As seen in Example 11, after the call-taker has collected information about the location in which the event has occurred and the type of event, the interrogative series is marked as completed ("okay") (Merritt, 1980; Mondada & Sorjonen, 2021), providing a link to the last phase of the call: that is, granting the request ("we'll send someone immediately", line 14). In general, after the request has been satisfied, the entire call draws quickly to a close, usually with a thank you from the caller (line 14: "thank you") (Nordberg, 1998).

The final (or 'distal', cf. Koole & van Burgsteden, 2022, p. 264) "thank you" is a display of appreciation through which "the callers portray themselves as the beneficiaries of the service provided by the call-taker on behalf of the organization" (Heritage & Clayman, 2010, p. 82). In the data discussed by Koole and van Burgsteden (2022, p. 260), around 80% of the calls ended with either the caller or the call-taker thanking the other. In fact, the final "thank you" can be also issued by call-takers, when the caller is recognized as presenting himself/herself as a good citizen concerned about issues of general interest (as when the caller rings to report an accident between two cars that she has witnessed: see Koole & van Burgsteden, 2022, p. 260).[32] Consider the following excerpt:

Excerpt 2.12 Thanks (from a Call to Police)

```
92 Ctaker      va bon occhei, ci mandiamo qualcuno a controllare.
               good, okay, we'll send someone to check.
93 Caller:     grazie. sa[lve
               thanks. bye
94 Ctaker                 [grazie, buongiorno.
                           thanks, have a good day.
95 Caller:     salve.
               bye.
```

[32] On expressions of caller satisfaction in calls between callers and cancer specialist nurses on a leading cancer helpline in the United Kingdom, see Woods et al. (2015).

In this call, the caller has rung the police to have a police officer inspect a suspicious package found lying on the ground in a car park (the beginning of this call is discussed in Chap. 3). In Excerpt 2.12, the call-taker has just granted deployment of the assistance requested by the caller (line 92), who expresses gratitude for the promise of intervention (line 93). At the same time, the call-taker expresses his gratitude to the caller (line 94) for his concern about issues of public interest.

The provision of the "thank you" is also prefiguring the end of the call. We have seen how emergency calls are brought to a close[33]: the provision of help and the promise of intervention are all that the callers were seeking, "such that the canonical four-part closings (in which parties deploy a round of passing tokens 'okay'—'okay', that display 'no mentionable to be mentioned' followed by a round of closing particles, 'bye'—'bye') are not relevant" (Raymond & Zimmerman, 2016, p. 732).

5 Problems of Communication

Things are not always so simple. Some studies[34] have shown that between caller and call-taker there can be an "interactional asynchrony" (Jefferson & Lee, 1981, p. 402) or problems in communication that may even give rise to serious practical problems (Whalen et al., 1988).

Consider the following example:

Excerpt 2.13 Send the Helicopter, Lines from 16 to 24—Continuing from Excerpt 2.9

```
19 Caller    °ma vaffanculo° ((heard in the background))
             fuck
20 Ctaker    sì mi dica.
             yes tell me.
21 Caller    mandate l'elicottero, non non non so.
             send the helicopter, I don't know.
```

(*continued*)

[33] On opening up closings in conversation see Schegloff and Sacks (1973).

[34] See for instance Whalen et al. (1988); Tracy (1997); Whalen and Zimmerman (1998); Tracy and Tracy (1998a, 1998b); Tracy (2002); Svennevig (2012); Perez-Gonzalez (1998).

Excerpt 2.13 (continued)

```
22 Ctaker    no, ascolti, lei non deve dirmi cosa devo mandare,
             no, listen, you don't have to say what I have to send
23           lei mi di[ca le condizioni della persona.
             tell me about the person's condition.
24 Caller              [(           )
25           signora, c'è un ragazzo che sta male qua.
             madam, there is a guy who is not feeling well here.
26 Ctaker    ecco. respira?
             okay. is he breathing?
27 Caller    sembra di no, sembra, cazzo!
             it seems not, it seems, fuck it!
28           ((a click is heard - caller ends the call))
29 Ctaker    mi dia il telefono per favore. (.) pronto?
             give me your phone number please. (.) hello?
```

This is the continuation of the call transcribed in Excerpt 2.9. When the caller returns to the phone, the situation does not appear to have changed in terms of the information available. The call-taker hears the caller come back on the line (an expletive can be heard in the background, line 19) and with an open question (line 20: "yes, tell me") invites the caller to give additional details concerning his request for the dispatch of an ambulance. The caller is still unable to provide a more accurate description of the event. Instead of providing details, the caller makes another request on the basis of what the call-taker had prefigured (line 21: "send the helicopter, I don't know"). The response is treated by the call-taker as another request. It seems clear that two different expectations are involved: the caller uses a 'service transaction' frame, the kind used to order goods in a service transaction, while the call-taker operated instead in a regime of public service (Whalen et al., 1988).[35] Similarly, Tracy (1997) talks about a clash between a 'customer service' frame and a 'public service' frame. The call-taker admonishes the caller and tries to return to the questioning frame (lines 22–23: "no, listen, you don't have to say what I have to send tell me

[35] For an analysis of the "disparity of expectations" in out-of-hours telephone calls between caller and doctors, see Drew (1998).

about the person's condition"). In a way, the caller tries to re-establish the boundary between lay and expert knowledge (Zimmerman, 1998, p. 104), in order to realign the appropriate institutional roles of each of the participants. The caller's response is a formulation of the problem that once again employs the format of the announcement (line 25: "madam, there is a guy who is not feeling well here") and adds no further elements to his previous formulation. At this point, the caller's turn can also be interpreted as a protest against an interrogation procedure that wastes time instead of providing the required help. The call-taker treats the caller's reply as an opportunity to return to the query format and tries to continue the interrogation series (line 26: "okay. is he breathing?"). The return to the interrogation format generates an angry and irritated response and an annoyed exclamation from the caller (line 27: "it seems not, it seems, fuck it!") and then the call is immediately closed. Although in this case an ambulance had already been sent by the call-taker to the machine shop of Vigarona (not indicated in the transcript—the ambulance was dispatched in between the two parts of the call), the call-taker was unable to obtain much more information about the event that had generated the emergency call before the call was abruptly closed. This is a case of 'unilateral termination' as described by Raymond and Zimmerman (2016, pp. 724–725).

This call is not only an example of a possible problem in emergency communications—that is, a mis-synchrony, a mis-alignment between the caller and the call-taker,[36] each with his/her own horizon of relevance—it is also an example of how emotions, 'rage' and 'hysteria', can be an important dimension of emergency moments and interfere with the implementation of professional help (Whalen & Zimmerman, 1998; Tracy & Tracy, 1998a, 1998b; Schuler, 2001; Paoletti, 2012; Garcia, 2013; Fele, 2014). From an interactional perspective, the call-taker's definition of a person as 'hysterical' does not amount to the recognition of a particular psychological state of the caller, but rather to a situated incompetence: the caller's inability to cooperate, during the call, in the accomplishment of the institutional tasks of the emergency organization (Whalen &

[36] For a case of resistance to comply achieved through the use of a category of person, see Berger et al. (2016). For the ways in which call-takers can be successful in persuading the caller to collaborate (in this case recruit a bystander to perform cardio-pulmonary resuscitation (CPR) until the ambulance arrive), see Riou et al. (2020).

Zimmerman, 1998:144). There is thus a kind of paradox at the root of emergency calls that can make them problematic. On the one hand, the more serious the event, the more necessary it seems to convey the perception of seriousness directly to the person who is institutionally in a position to provide the help—the open expression of feelings (Mauss, 1921; Goffman, 1978) being in some cultures the way to react to distressing situations, making it possible for observers to infer the seriousness of the event. On the other hand, however, the open expression of feelings prevents the establishment of a collaborative stance, and it can be a real obstacle to the collection of information and to the definition of the appropriate response in these specific stressful circumstances (Whalen & Zimmerman, 1998, p. 150).

6 Conclusions

We have seen in this brief presentation the subtle practical ways in which calls arriving at a public safety answering point are managed by call-takers. The call-takers receive the calls from citizens and manage to collect the relevant information that they will transmit to the dispatchers so that they can send help to the site. The operators of the public safety answering points are trained professionally: but frequently what is prescribed in manuals and in protocols has very little to do with what happens in the real management of emergency calls. Interaction research is thus able to document and make evident the good practices that are the routinized procedures regularly employed by operators, often against the prescriptions of the conventional procedures. Such studies have interesting implications for professional practice in dealing with emergency calls: conversation analysis utilizes a methodical procedure, based on sequential principles, in order to uncover the granular aspects (Schegloff, 2000) that constitute the normal, competent activity of dealing with emergency calls. Conversation analysis provides an analytical system for recognizing, describing, analysing and defining this swarm of practical skills embedded in professional work. A few years ago, Gilsinan (1989, p. 342) pointed out, with reference to the American 911 emergency number, that it was necessary to take into consideration two aspects of emergency operations: "focusing externally, [operators] can improve the quality of incoming data. Working with citizens, upgrading equipment, and training operators on how on elicit better detail from callers are some of the strategies that flow from this organizational perspective. Administrator should also focus inward, however. Organizational quasi-theories embedded in codes, manuals, and employees' assumptions about tasks may negate any effects of 'better' data. Meaningful data (i.e. information), not better data, is what binds an organization and its clients." This book is an invitation to look at what call-takers and callers actually do, and an encouragement to set aside any previous theory about what they do. Instead of focusing on what they should do according to protocols and manuals, it urges researchers to pay attention to what really happens in genuine situations.

Other aspects of emergency calls are examined in the following chapters.

References

Albert, S., Housley, W., & Stokoe, E. (2019). In case of emergency, order pizza. An urgent case of action formation and recognition. In *1st International Conference on Conversational User Interfaces (CUI 2019)*, August 22–23, 2019, Dublin, Ireland. ACM, New York. https://doi.org/10.1145/3342775.3342800

Arminen, I., & Leinonen, M. (2006). Mobile phone call openings: Tailoring answers to personalized summonses. *Discourse Studies, 8*(3), 339–368.

Berdowski, J., Beekhuis, F., Zwinderman, A. H., Tijssen, J. G., & Koster, R. W. (2009). Importance of the first link: Description and recognition of an out-of-hospital cardiac arrest in an emergency call. *Circulation, 119*(15), 2096–2102.

Berger, I., Kitzinger, C., & Ellis, S. J. (2016). Using a category to accomplish resistance in the context of an emergency call: Michael Jackson's doctor. *Pragmatics, 26*(4), 563–582.

Bergmann, J. R. (1992). Alarmiertes Verstehen: Kommunikation in Feuerwehrnotrufen. In T. Jung & S. Müller-Doohm (Eds.), *"Wirklichkeit" im Deutungsprozeß. Verstehen und Methoden in den Kultur- und Sozialwissenschaften* (pp. 283–328). Suhrkamp.

Clayman, S. E., & Heritage, J. (2014). Benefactor and beneficiaries. In P. Drew & E. Couper-Kuhlen (Eds.), *Requesting in social interaction* (pp. 55–86). John Benjamins.

Craven, A., & Potter, J. (2010). Directives: Entitlement and contingency in action. *Discourse Studies, 12*(4), 419–442.

Cromdal, J., Landqvist, H., Persson-Thunqvist, D., & Osvaldsson, K. (2012). Finding out what's happened: Two procedures for opening emergency calls. *Discourse Studies, 14*(4), 371–397.

Cromdal, J., Persson-Thunqvist, D., & Osvaldsson, K. (2012). "SOS 112 what has occurred?" Managing openings in children's emergency calls. *Discourse, Context & Media, 1*(4), 183–202.

Curl, T. S., & Drew, P. (2008). Contingency and action: A comparison of two forms of requesting. *Research on Language and Social Interaction, 41*(2), 129–153.

Danby, S., Baker, C., & Emmison, M. (2005). Four observations on openings in calls to kids help line. In C. D. Baker, M. Emmison, & A. Firth (Eds.), *Calling for help. Language and social interaction in telephone helplines* (pp. 133–151). Benjamins.

Deppermann, A., & Gubina, A. (2021). Positionally-sensitive action-ascription: Uses of Kannst du X? 'Can you X?' in their sequential and multimodal context. *Interactional Linguistics, 1*(2), 183–215.

Drew, P. (1998). Out of hours calls to the doctor: Misalignment between callers and doctor during diagnostic questioning. In S. Cmejrkova, J. Hoffmannová, O. Müllerová, & J. Světlá (Eds.), *Dialoganalyse VI/2: Referate der 6. Arbeitstagung, Prag 1996* (pp. 65–78). Max Niemeyer Verlag.

Drew, P., & Couper-Kuhlen, E. (2014). Requesting—From speech act to recruitment. In P. Drew & E. Couper-Kuhlen (Eds.), *Requesting in social interaction* (pp. 1–34). John Benjamins.

Drew, P., & Heritage, J. (1992). Talk at work: An introduction. In P. Drew & J. Heritage (Eds.), *Talk at work: Interaction in institutional settings* (pp. 3–65). Cambridge University Press.

Drew, P., & Walker, T. (2010). Citizen's emergency calls to police: Requesting assistance in calls to the police. In M. Coulthard & A. Johnson (Eds.), *Handbook of forensic linguistic* (pp. 95–110). Routledge.

Emmison, M., & Danby, S. (2007). "Who's the friend in the background?": Interactional strategies in determining authenticity in calls to a national children's helpline. *Australian Review of Applied Linguistics, 30*(3), 31–31.

Fele, G. (2014). Stati interni e cognizione: che cosa facciamo quando parliamo con qualcuno. In L. Muzzetto (Ed.), *Wittgenstein e il pensiero sociologico* (pp. 189–212). Pisa.

Fox, B. A., & Heinemann, T. (2021). Are they requests? An exploration of declaratives of trouble in service encounters. *Research on Language and Social Interaction, 54*(1), 20–38.

Fussell, P. (2002). *Uniforms. Why we are what we wear.* Houghton Mifflin.

Garcia, A. C. (2013). Problematic emergency service calls. In A. C. Garcia (Ed.), *An introduction to interaction. Understanding talk in formal and informal settings* (pp. 166–182). Bloomsbury.

Garcia, A. C. (2015). 'Something really weird has happened': Losing the 'big picture' in emergency service calls. *Journal of Pragmatics, 84*, 102–120.

Garcia, A. C. (2022). A preliminary investigation of the use of racial/ethnic categories in emergency telephone calls in the United States. *Journal of Applied Communication Research, 50*(4), 345–362.

Garcia, A. C., & Parmer, P. A. (1999). Misplaced mistrust: The collaborative construction of doubt in 911 emergency calls. *Symbolic Interaction, 22*(4), 297–324.

Gilsinan, J. F. (1989). They is clowning tough: 911 and the social construction of reality. *Criminology, 27*(2), 329–344.

Goffman, E. (1978). Response cries. *Language, 54*(4), 787–815.

González-Martínez, E. (2017). Ouverture d'appels téléphoniques infirmière-transporteur à l'hôpital. *Revue française de linguistique appliquée, 22*(2), 165–183.

González-Martínez, E., & Drew, P. (2021). Informings as recruitment in nurses' intrahospital telephone calls. *Journal of Pragmatics, 186*, 48–59.

Heritage, J., & Clayman, S. E. (2010). Calls for emergency service. In J. Heritage & S. Clayman (Eds.), *Talk in action: Interactions, identities, and institutions* (pp. 53–100). Wiley-Blackwell.

Imbens-Bailey, A., & McCabe, A. (2000). The discourse of distress: A narrative analysis of emergency calls to 911. *Language and Communication, 20*, 275–296.

Jefferson, G., & Lee, J. R. E. (1981). The rejection of advice: Managing the problematic convergence of a 'troubles-telling' and a 'service encounter'. *Journal of Pragmatics, 5*(5), 399–422.

Kent, A., & Antaki, C. (2020). Police call-takers' first substantive question projects the outcome of the call. *Applied Linguistics, 41*(5), 640–661.

Kevoe-Feldman, H., & Sutherland, C. B. (2018). The "four-second rule" for identifying the active silent 911 caller. *Annals of Emergency Dispatch & Response, 6*(1), 5–9.

Koole, T., & van Burgsteden, L. (2022). Actions and identities in emergency calls: The case of thanking. In A. Deppermann & M. Haugh (Eds.), *Action ascription in interaction* (pp. 256–276). Cambridge University Press.

Koole, T., & Verberg, N. (2017). Aligning caller and call-taker: The opening phrase of Dutch emergency calls. *Pragmatics and Society, 8*(1), 129–153.

Landgren, J., & Bergstrand, F. (2010). Mobile live video in emergency response: Its use and consequences. *Bulletin of the American Society for Information Science and Technology, 36*(5), 27–29.

Larsen, T. (2013). Dispatching emergency assistance: Callers' claims of entitlement and call takers' decisions. *Research on Language and Social Interaction, 46*(3), 205–230.

Leydon, G. M., Ekberg, K., & Drew, P. (2013). "How can I help?" Nurse call openings on a cancer helpline and implications for call progressivity. *Patient Education and Counseling, 92*(1), 23–30.

Mauss, M. (1921). L'expression obligatoire des sentiments (rituels oraux funéraires australiens). *Journal de psychologie, 18*, 425–434.

Meehan, A. J. (1989). Assessing the "police-worthiness" of citizen complaints to the police: Accountability and the negotiation of "facts". In D. T. Helm, W. T. Anderson, A. J. Meehan, & A. Rawls (Eds.), *The interactional order: New directions in the study of social order* (pp. 116–140). Irvington Publishers, Inc.

Mellinger, W. M. (1992). Talk-as-work: The case of paramedic calls for emergency field orders. *Current Research on Occupations and Professions, 7*, 79–109.

Merritt, M. (1980). On the use of OK in service encounters. In E. W. Shuy & A. Shunkal (Eds.), *Language use and the uses of language* (pp. 162–172). Georgetown University Press.

Mondada, L., & Sorjonen, M.-L. (2021). OKAY in closings and transitions. In E. Betz, A. Deppermann, L. Mondada, & M.-L. Sorjonen (Eds.), *OKAY across languages: Toward a comparative approach to its use in talk-in-interaction* (pp. 94–127). John Benjamins.

Monzoni, C. M. (2009a). Direct complaints in (Italian) calls to the ambulance: The use of negatively framed questions. *Journal of Pragmatics, 41*(12), 2465–2478.

Monzoni, C. M. (2009b). Preference organization and complaining in (Italian) 118 emergency calls to the ambulance. *Dialogue Analysis, XI*, 249–261.

Monzoni, C., & Zorzi, D. (2003). Le telefonate d'emergenza: un confronto fra l'italiano e l'inglese. In E. M. Thüne & S. Leonardi (Eds.), *Telefonare in diverse lingue. Organizzazione sequenziale, routine e rituali in telefonate di servizio, di emergenza e fàtiche*. FrancoAngeli.

Neustaedter, C., Jones, B., O'Hara, K., & Sellen, A. (2017). An analysis of next generation 9-1-1: Video calling for emergency situations. *Connections Lab Technical Report 2017-0920-01*, Simon Fraser University.

Neustaedter, C., McGee, J., & Dash, P. (2019). Sharing 9-1-1 video call information between dispatchers and firefighters during everyday emergencies. In *Proceedings of the 2019 on Designing Interactive Systems Conference* (pp. 567–580).

Nordberg, B. (1998). On closings in alarm calls. *Sprak och Stil, 8*, 65–103.

Palma, E., Antonaci, D., Colì, A., & Cicolini, G. (2014). Analysis of emergency medical services triage and dispatch errors by registered nurses in Italy. *Journal of Emergency Nursing, 40*(5), 476–483.

Paoletti, I. (2012). Operators managing callers' sense of urgency in calls to the medical emergency number. *Pragmatics, 22*(4), 671–695.

Penn, C., Koole, T., & Nattrass, R. (2017). When seconds count: A study of communication variables in the opening segment of emergency calls. *Journal of Health Psychology, 22*(10), 1256–1264.

Perera, N., Riou, M., Ball, S., Birnie, T., Morgan, A., Whiteside, A., Bailey, P., & Finn, J. (2020). The trajectory of repairs in the defibrillator sequence during emergency cardiac arrest calls–balancing progressivity and intersubjectivity. *Communication and Medicine, 17*(2), 150–164.

Perez-Gonzalez, L. (1998). The conversational dynamics of interactional dispute in conflictive calls for emergency assistance: A single case study. In A. Sanchez-Macarro & R. Carter (Eds.), *Linguistic choice across genres: Variation in spoken and written English* (pp. 265–290). John Benjamins.

Raymond, G., & Zimmerman, D. H. (2007). Rights and responsibilities in calls for help: The case of the Mountain Glade Fire. *Research on Language and Social Interaction, 40*(1), 33–61.

Raymond, G., & Zimmerman, D. H. (2016). Closing matters: Alignment and misalignment in sequence and call closings in institutional interaction. *Discourse Studies, 18*(6), 1–34.

Reiter, R. M. (2006). Interactional closeness in service calls to a Montevidean carer service company. *Research on Language and Social Interaction, 39*(1), 7–39.

Riou, M., Ball, S., Williams, T. A., Whiteside, A., O'Halloran, K. L., Bray, J., Perkins, G. D., Smith, K., Cameron, P., Fatovich, D. M., & Inoue, M. (2017). 'Tell me exactly what's happened': When linguistic choices affect the efficiency of emergency calls for cardiac arrest. *Resuscitation, 117*, 58–65.

Riou, M., Ball, S., O'Halloran, K. L., Whiteside, A., Williams, T. A., & Finn, J. (2018). Hijacking the dispatch protocol: When callers pre-empt their reason-for-the-call in emergency calls about cardiac arrest. *Discourse Studies, 20*(5), 666–687.

Riou, M., Ball, S., Williams, T. A., Whiteside, A., Cameron, P., Fatovich, D. M., Perkins, G. D., Smith, K., Bray, J., Inoue, M., Halloran, K. L., Bailey, P., Brink, D., & Finn, J. (2018). 'She's sort of breathing': What linguistic factors determine call-taker recognition of agonal breathing in emergency calls for cardiac arrest? *Resuscitation, 122*, 92–98.

Riou, M., Ball, S., Whiteside, A., Gallant, S., Morgan, A., Bailey, P., & Finn, J. (2020). Caller resistance to perform cardio-pulmonary resuscitation in emergency calls for cardiac arrest. *Social Science & Medicine, 256*, 113045.

Schegloff, E. A. (1968). Sequencing in conversational openings. *American Anthropologist, 70*(6), 1075–1095.

Schegloff, E. A. (1979). Identification and recognition in telephone conversation openings. In G. Psathas (Ed.), *Everyday language: Studies in ethnomethodology* (pp. 23–78). Irvington Publishers, Inc.

Schegloff, E. A. (1986). The routine as achievement. *Human Studies, 9*(2–3), 111–151.

Schegloff, E. A. (2000). On granularity. *Annual Review of Sociology, 26*, 715–720.

Schegloff, E. A. (2002a). Beginnings in the telephone. In J. E. Katz & M. Aakhus (Eds.), *Perpetual contact: Mobile communication, private talk, public performance* (pp. 284–300). Cambridge University Press.

Schegloff, E. A. (2002b). Reflections on research on telephone conversation: Issues of cross-cultural scope and scholarly exchange, interactional import and consequences. In L. Kang Kwong & P. Theodossia-Soula (Eds.), *Telephone calls: Unity and diversity in conversational structure across languages and cultures* (pp. 249–281). John Benjamins.

Schegloff, E. A., & Sacks, H. (1973). Opening up closings. *Semiotica, 8*(4), 289–327.

Schuler, S. (2001). Talking community at 911: The centrality of communication in coping with emotional labour. In G. J. Shepered & E. W. Rothenbuhler (Eds.), *Communication and community* (pp. 53–77). Lawrence Erlbaum.

Sharrock, W. W., & Turner, R. (1978). On a conversational environment for equivocality. In J. N. Schenkein (Ed.), *Studies in the organization of conversational interaction* (pp. 173–197). Academic Press.

Sorjonen, M.-L., Raevaara, L., & Couper-Kuhlen, E. (Eds.). (2017). *Imperative turns at talk: The design of directives in action*. John Benjamins.

Stivers, T., & Rossano, F. (2010). Mobilizing response. *Research on Language and Social Interaction, 43*(1), 3–31.

Svennevig, J. (2012). On being heard in emergency calls. The development of hostility in a fatal emergency call. *Journal of Pragmatics, 44*(11), 1393–1412.

Svensson, M., & Hällgren, M. (2018). Sensemaking in sensory deprived settings: The role of non-verbal auditory cues for emergency assessment. *European Management Journal, 36*(3), 306–318.

Taleghani-Nikazm, C., Betz, E., & Golato, P. (Eds.). (2020). *Mobilizing others: Grammar and lexis within larger activities*. John Benjamins.

Tennent, E. (2021). "I'm calling in regard to my son": Entitlement obligation and opportunity to seek help for others. *British Journal of Social Psychology, 60*(3), 870–887.

Tennent, E., & Weatherall, A. (2019). Disclosing violence in calls for help. *Gender and Language, 13*(2), 270–288.

Tracy, K. (1997). Interactional trouble in emergency service requests: A problem of frames. *Research on Language and Social Interaction, 30*(4), 315–343.

Tracy, S. J. (2002). When questioning turns to face threat: An interactional sensitivity in 911 call-taking. *Western Journal of Communication, 66*(2), 129–157.

Tracy, K., & Agne, R. R. (2002). 'I just need to ask somebody some questions': Sensitivities in domestic dispute calls. In J. Cotterill (Ed.), *Language in the legal process* (pp. 75–90). Palgrave.

Tracy, K., & Anderson, D. L. (1999). Relational positioning strategies in police calls: A dilemma. *Discourse Studies, 1*(2), 201–225.

Tracy, K., & Tracy, S. J. (1998a). Rudeness at 911: Reconceptualizing face and face attack. *Human Communication Research, 25*(2), 225–251.

Tracy, S. J., & Tracy, K. (1998b). Emotion labor at 911: A case study and theoretical critique. *Journal of Applied Communication Research, 26*(4), 390–411.

Vaajala, T., Arminen, I., & De Rycker, A. (2013). Misalignments in Finnish emergency call openings: Legitimacy, asymmetries and multi-tasking as interactional contests. In A. De Rycker & Z. Mohd Don (Eds.), *Discourse and crisis: Critical perspectives* (pp. 131–157). John Benjamins.

Vinkhuyzen, E., Whalen, M., & Szymanski, M. (2006). Security, efficiency, and customer service in calls to a financial services organization. *Revue française de linguistique appliquée, 11*(2), 53–68.

Wakin, M. A., & Zimmerman, D. H. (1999). Reduction and specialization in emergency and directory assistance calls. *Research on Language and Social Interaction, 32*(4), 409–437.

Weatherall, A., Danby, S., Osvaldsson, K., Cromdal, J., & Emmison, M. (2016). Pranking in children's helpline calls. *Australian Journal of Linguistics, 36*(2), 224–238.

Whalen, M. R., & Zimmerman, D. H. (1987). Sequential and institutional contexts in calls for help. *Social Psychology Quarterly, 50*(2), 172–185.

Whalen, M. R., & Zimmerman, D. H. (1990). Describing trouble: Practical epistemology in citizen calls to the police. *Language in Society, 19*(4), 465–492.

Whalen, J., & Zimmerman, D. H. (1998). Observations on the display and management of emotion in naturally occurring activities: The case of "hysteria" in calls to 9-1-1. *Social Psychology Quarterly, 61*(2), 141–159.

Whalen, J., Zimmerman, D. H., & Whalen, M. (1988). When words fail: A single case analysis. *Social Problems, 35*(4), 335–362.

Wilson, T. P. (1991). Social structure and the sequential organization of interaction. In D. Boden & D. H. Zimmerman (Eds.), *Talk and social structure: Studies in ethnomethodology and conversation analysis* (pp. 22–43). Polity Press.

Woods, C. J., Drew, P., & Leydon, G. M. (2015). Closing calls to a cancer helpline: Expressions of caller satisfaction. *Patient Education and Counselling, 98*(8), 943–953.

Zimmerman, D. H. (1984). Talk and its occasions: The case of calling the police. In D. Schiffrin (Ed.), *Meaning, form, and use in context: Linguistic applications. Georgetown University roundtable on language and linguistics* (pp. 210–228). Georgetown University Press.

Zimmerman, D. H. (1992a). Achieving context: Openings in emergency calls. In G. Watson & R. M. Seiler (Eds.), *Text in context: Contributions to ethnomethodology* (pp. 35–51). Sage.

Zimmerman, D. H. (1992b). The interactional organization of calls for emergency assistance. In P. Drew & J. Heritage (Eds.), *Talk at work: Social interaction in institutional settings* (pp. 418–469). Cambridge University Press.

Zimmerman, D. H. (1998). Identity, context and interaction. In C. Antaki & S. Widdicombe (Eds.), *Identities in talk* (pp. 87–106). Sage.

CHAPTER 3

The Search for a Place

Abstract This chapter examines in detail phase 3 of the telephone call: that is, collection of information by the call-taker. In this phase, there are two kinds of basic information that the call-taker must collect: first, what has happened; second, where it has happened. The former aspect, in terms of the way in which the problem is formulated in the call, has been briefly examined in the previous chapter. The latter, which is the way in which the place of the emergency may be formulated, is the topic of this chapter.

Keywords Place formulation • Emergency location • Locating work • Common sense geography • Landmarks

1 How to Locate the Scene of an Emergency

Positioning an event in a particular location is a typical task that emergency operators must carry out at the dispatch centre.[1] The operators work in control centres, which are centralized units that handle emergency calls from sometimes remote places. Dispatch centres must control events that are distant in space. Deciding where exactly these events are located is

[1] It is true that technological improvements in handling emergency calls (with mapping and location information) can have consequences in the ways the call-takers design their questions about location (Kevoe-Feldman, 2019).

G. Fele, *Emergency Communication*,
https://doi.org/10.1007/978-3-031-26239-5_3

a crucial task when dealing with emergencies. But, at the same time, prompt action is essential. Determining where an event generating an emergency has happened is important in order to choose which emergency station should be alerted (from which place or town the ambulance should be sent; in what direction; which emergency station is nearest to the place of the emergency) and to be able to 'guess' what general kind of emergency may be ongoing (if the call is from a care home or a motorway, for instance, can orient the call-taker's attention immediately to a broad set of very different emergencies). But at the same time, the response should be fast. There are in place two conflicting demands of an emergency response: on the one hand, the response should be fast, but based on accurate information; on the other, obtaining accurate information takes time and impinges on the progressivity of the call.

In this chapter, I examine only the search for the location of an emergency in the telephone calls, as a matter involving the caller and the call-taker. In fact, the descriptions and formulations of places by callers are not the only resource which the operators can use in order to decide where an emergency is located. The work of establishing 'where it has happened' in an emergency call centre is much more complicated. The operators in the operation room can use several instruments and supports—in electronic or paper form: information systems, maps, cartographies and so on (Mondada, 2010, 2011a, 2011b). Moreover, these technological supports are rendered meaningful through a complex web of social interaction and collaboration among the people working in the dispatch centre (Pettersson, 2001). For example, the call-taker can receive occasional help in recognizing a place from colleagues who are working in other rooms and are not working on the same critical event, but who are familiar with the places being talked about (and aloud) in the operation room (Pettersson, 2001). In the dispatch centre that I examined, there were two 'rooms' to which the emergency telephone calls arrived. Each room dealt with calls coming from only a part of the area. Some operators preferred to work in one room rather than in the other, because of the 'local knowledge' (Normark & Randall, 2005) that they could show regarding the physical, geographic, orographic, topological and so on, characteristics of the territory covered in that particular room. In this chapter, I will not take any account of this complex social interaction in the room. Moreover, what might be interesting but is not examined here is the process whereby information about the place which the call-taker can elicit from the caller is transposed into a format suitable for the actual dispatch. In the context studied, the call-taker logged the 'data' obtained in the phone call on an electronic form only after the call had concluded. During the phone call, relevant information was recorded by the call-taker with a pen and paper. Often, the electronic form was filled up only after the completion of the call. How the information was categorized in order to be accepted by the system was a major issue in the organizational management of the dispatch centre.[2] The way in which the system constituted a constraint and/or a resource in the work of the operators is another important analytical issue.[3] Furthermore, the dispatcher in his/her work provided instructions to the ambulance crews on 'where the event has happened'. How the dispatch was made and the ways in which the original information about places was translated into the dispatch format warrant analysis.[4] Last but not least, monitoring of the progress of the ambulance's journey is another interesting part of the job of the operators which is relevant to analysis of place names. The crews on the ground can 'know better' than the dispatcher in the control room the places and the geography mentioned in the emergency call. Hence, there may be a third form of 'local knowledge', which is displayed by the crews at the moment when they are called into action. The acquaintance of the crews with the area can let them consider as 'specific' and 'particular' (i.e., recognizable for all practical purposes) a place description that for the operators has only 'generic' and 'vague' features. At the same time, very interesting cases arise and can be analysed when the crew has some kind of difficulty in recognizing the right place to go to, or occasions when the ambulance 'gets lost'. The ways in which "bona-fide members of a collectivity" (ten Have, 2002) analyse these 'states of displacement' are a 'gold mine' for analysts of the interactional and conversational ways in which formulations of places are shaped.

This chapter is aware of the complexity of place characterization during an emergency, but it focuses only on the ways in which places are described in telephone calls requesting assistance or help. In these cases, the location of a place and its recognizability by the parties is an interactional work integral to talk. The caller has only the words at hand with which to enable the call-taker to recognize and to characterize a place. The call-taker relies on conversational strategies in order to elicit recognizable descriptions of places.

[2] On categorization of the emergencies, see Greco (2004) and Rollet (2015); on categorization of people, see Kameo and Whalen (2015).

[3] On how computer tools and information systems are utilized by the call-takers (not necessarily of an emergency call and dispatch centre) and how the typing on the keyboard impinges on the production of talk, see Frankel (1989); Heath and Luff (2000); Houtkoop et al. (2005); Mondada (2010; 2011a); Nattrass et al. (2017); Rollet (2013); Whalen (1995a, 1995b); Kameo and Whalen (2015).

[4] See Chap. 6 for an analysis of how dispatches are done.

2 Place Formulation

That the formulation of the place occupies a large part of the concerns of the caller (as a normative dimension to which both parties are oriented) can be seen in the initial sequence of the telephone call, at the very beginning of the caller's turn. The definition of the place of the emergency is one of the first tasks to which the caller is oriented. If we consider the sequential ordering of calls, we see that in many of them the definition of the place of the event generating the request for intervention occupies the very first part of the telephone call, even before the formulation of the problem.[5] We know that the positioning of an element (or elements) in the sequence and the construction of the speaker's turn is not a neutral aspect of the conversational interaction; rather, it can convey normative orientations of the parties towards something that they feel should be stated as soon possible (for instance, agreements are made in the very next turn, without delay, while disagreements are deferred to a later place in the turn or to subsequent turns) (Pomerantz & Heritage, 2013). We have seen how emergency telephone calls are organized in ways that allow the formulation of the reason for the call in the first possible point of the sequence. The first turn of the caller (containing a request for assistance) usually comprises two main components: one is constituted by formulation of 'something happened'; the second is constituted by formulation of 'where this something happened'. One is the formulation of trouble, that is, a report, description or narrative account of some problematic event or situation. The other is some kind of formulation of place.

Often, this 'place formulation' is given even before the formulation of the fact that generated the request for assistance (Nattrass et al., 2017). This is the very first slot in which the caller can have his/her turn:

[5] It has been noted that a common feature of mobile phone conversations is the giving of a geographical formulation as part of the opening sequence of a phone call. See Mondada (2011a, pp. 396–398); Laurier (2001); Arminen (2006); Relieu (2002). In general, mobile phones appear to be very useful in rapidly reporting emergencies (Chapman & Schofield, 1998), while at the same time placing pressure on call and dispatch centres because of the growing fear and anxieties of these times among the population (Eriksson, 2010). See also Landgren and Nulden (2007) and Ludwig et al. (2013).

Excerpt 3.1 Cyclist Fallen Down a Ravine

01	Ctaker	centodiciotto? *one one eight?*
02	Caller	(-monte rovere) ascolti, al- al monte Rovere, *(-monte rovere) listen, at- at monte Rovere,*
03		chilometro dicio- e:[:h[nove==nove, *kilometre eight- e:[:h[nine==nine*
04		è caduto uno in bicicletta giù da un burrone. *a cyclist has fallen down a ravine.*

Excerpt 3.2 Accident on the Motorway

01	Ctaker	centodiciotto? *one one eight?*
02	Caller	signora, sono sull'autostrada e da CITTA 1 *madam, I'm on the motorway and from CITY 1*
03		(stiamo andando) verso CITTA 2. *(we're heading) toward TOWN 2.*
04		c'è stato un incidente. *there has been an accident.*

Excerpt 3.3 Motorbike Accident

01	Ctaker	centodiciotto *one one eight*
02	Caller	pronto *hello*
03	Ctaker	pronto *hello*
04	Caller	pronto, guardi strada della LOCALITA? *hello, listen road of LOCAL PLACE?*
05	Ctaker	sì *yes*
06	Caller	c'è stato un incidente, *there has been an accident,*
07		mi è venuto dietro u- una moto, *a motorbike has crashed into the back of my car*

Excerpt 3.4 A Plane Just Crashed

```
01 Ctaker   sì, Verona emergenza?
            yes, Verona emergency?
02 Caller   eh, hem, in località, Poiane, in via Dossobuono,
            eh, ehm, in the Poiane countryside, Dossobuono Road
03          a Sommacampagna, è appena caduto un aereo.
            Sommacampagna, a plane has just crashed.
```

In all four transcripts, the typical format for delivery of the reason for the call seems to be: [formulation of place] + [formulation of the event]. The formulation of place appears to occupy the very first opportunity to talk, the very first part of the first turn by the caller. In a sense, formulation of the place seems to be more compelling upon the caller, even more than the same formulation of the event that generates the request for intervention (even in the case of a 'big event' emergency, e.g. a disaster as in Excerpt 3.4) (Bolaños-Carpio, 2021).

That this pattern exhibits a shared orientation by the parties—that is, one that is not just an orientation by the caller alone—is apparent on occasions when the formulation of the event precedes any formulation of the place (Mondada, 2011a, p. 398)[6]:

Excerpt 3.5 Screwdriver into Hand

```
01 Ctaker   centodiciotto pronto
            one one eight hello
      ((1 line omitted))
03 Caller   pronto
            hello
04 Ctaker   sì mi dica
            yes, tell me
05 Caller   'scolta mio figlio si è piantato cacciavite
            listen my son has stuck a screwdriver
06          nella mano sinistra, cosa devo farle?
            into his left hand, what must I do?
07 Ctaker   ma e: da dove chiama, scusi?
            but e: where are you calling from, sorry?
```

[6] Kent and Antaki (2020) note that requests for the caller's location by the call-taker in the first substantive question are treated as indicating that emergency action will be taken.

Excerpt 3.6 Can You Bring an Ambulance

```
01 Ctaker   centodiciotto?
            one one eight?
02 Caller   buongiorno mi può portare subito un'autoambulanza
            good morning can you quickly bring an ambulance
03 Ctaker   dove?
            where?
04 Caller   a CITTA in NOME VIA trentacinque
            to TOWN STREET NAME thirty five
05 Ctaker   NOME VIA?
            STREET NAME?
06 Caller   sì
            yes
07 Ctaker   trentacinque
            thirty five
08 Caller   sì. è la NOME AZIENDA, è un'azienda
            yes. it's the FIRM NAME, it's a firm
09 Ctaker   NOME AZIENDA.
            FIRM NAME.
10 Caller   sì
            yes
11          (0.5)
12 Ctaker   cos'è successo?
            what's happened?
```

In Excerpt 3.5, the caller is using her first opportunity to talk (lines 5–6) to state the reason for her call, but only formulates a description of the event. In Excerpt 3.6, the caller makes only a request (line 2). In both cases, a kind of 'repair procedure' (Hayashi et al., 2013) is enacted by the call-taker. To move the interrogative series forward, and to begin the work of ascertaining the reason for the call, the call-taker first asks 'where' questions (3.5, line 7: *from where are you calling*; 3.6, line 3: *where* [do you need an ambulance]). Instead of determining what has happened, following what the caller said in his/her previous turn, the call-taker asks first a 'where-question', the required answer to which is a kind of place formulation on the caller's part (Nattrass et al., 2017, p. 74). Only after some kind of place formulation has been provided is the caller allowed to provide the description or give the report on the case.

So far, I have wanted to identify only what could be the first opportunity to provide a place description in an emergency call in the corpus that I studied. I have shown that these data exhibit a marked pattern of place formulation in the caller's very first opportunity to talk, and it occupies the first part of the first turn to talk. This evidences the salience of place formulation in emergency calls. Obviously, this is not the only sequential point in which formulation of the place of the event appears. As we shall see later, there are other points in an emergency telephone call where the call-taker resumes the work of determining 'where it happened'. For now, I shall shift from the issue of the 'position' of place formulation to the issue of the composition of this turn.

3 Descriptions of Places and 'Locating Work'

This chapter analyses in particular the 'locating work' by the parties during an emergency call. Referring to the seminal work by Emanuel Schegloff (1972, p. 81), we can state the problem of (place) description thus:

> The 'problem' of locational formulation is this: For any location to which reference is made, there is a set of terms each of which, by a correspondence test, is a correct way to refer to it. On any actual occasion of use, however, not any member of the set is 'right'. How is it that on particular occasions of use some term from the set is selected and other terms are rejected? [...] I seek to direct attention to the sorts of considerations that enter into the selection of a particular locational formulation, and the work a hearer does in analyzing its use.

Schegloff (1972, p. 106) writes that "in the selection and adequate hearing of a locational formulation, at least three orders of consideration are relevant: a location analysis, a membership analysis, and a topic analysis", that is, the activity being performed in an utterance. Emergency telephone calls have been examined in regard to the ways in which caller and answerer display an alignment of relevant identities as a requester of help and its dispatcher (Whalen & Zimmerman, 1987; Zimmerman, 1992a, 1992b, 1998), as we saw in Chap. 1. Furthermore, the turn of the caller can be inspected in order to see how it accomplishes the activity of reporting a problem or requesting assistance. For these reasons, in this chapter I shall leave aside considerations about membership analysis and topic analysis, to focus instead on location analysis by the parties. Schegloff states: "the selection of a location formulation requires of a speaker (and will exhibit for a hearer) an analysis of his own location and the location of his co-conversationalist(s), and of the objects whose location is being formulated (if that object is not one of the co-conversationalists)" (Schegloff, 1972, p. 83).

I shall only briefly discuss the activity being accomplished in a place description during an emergency call. Making a description is not a disinterested activity in an emergency telephone call. In the first instance, the caller must specify 'an exact' place, not a 'generic' and 'vague' one. Second, call-takers and callers are oriented to characterizing concrete, specific places, potentially recognizable to each other, for the purpose of the call, which is to receive help and assistance, and so that someone who is far away can reach the place concerned.[7] A description has a function. A description is not made to describe a state of the world, but to be used, that is, made recognizable. If an ambulance crew enters an area unknown to it, the crew must be able to recognize places and find the way (Mondada, 2011a). The description of places serves this institutional purpose (the description of some characteristics of a building, like its colour or shape, is not made in order to render its 'aesthetic qualities' visible).

To some extent, we can characterize the work of formulating a place with the Gestalt metaphor of "extracting an animal from the foliage" (Garfinkel, 2022, pp. 118–119). The task of recognizing a place from a description is similar to the perceptive game where one has to recognize a figure (an 'animal') which is hidden in a field ('foliage'). The task of the caller is to render visible and recognizable, only through his/her talk, the animal in the foliage. The interactional work of the caller and the call-taker is that of introducing and describing a *figure* that stands out from an undifferentiated and un-thematized *background*. The conversational work by the callers and call-takers consists in providing through their talk those particulars and those descriptions that convey salient aspects of the world—that is, which can render them recognizable to both of them.[8]

[7] See Haddington and Keisanen (2009), and Kazemi (2020), for studies on the negotiation of route to be taken and the shared recognizabilty of the place references.

[8] Crabtree et al. (2006) speak of "articulation work".

There are two basic methods in the management of emergency calls for the identification of places. One is collecting basic information which can be recorded as the 'official place' of the emergency—that is, the information which will be inserted into the information system and which will provide the 'official record' of the call, for all organizational purposes. These are basic formulations of places based on a few geographical coordinates or 'intrinsic' characterizations of places (names of places or 'G terms', in Schegloff's terminology (1992, p. 97)). The second is collecting more substantial information about both 'where that place is' and 'how to get there', using topological relations and relative references (Rm 'relation to members', Rl 'relation to landmark' and Rn 'place name' in Schegloff's terminology (1992, pp. 97–102)). In both cases, co-locating an object within a certain space means putting this object into an immediate containing region. Localizing an object and determining its location involves processes of dividing a space into sub-regions or segmenting it so as to 'narrow in' on an object's immediate environment. In the former case, the localization work is done through 'official' and formal definitions of places, whereas in the latter case it is accomplished through a work of relational positioning of the main reference vis-à-vis other reference points in the field. In the former case, the formulation of place rarely produces a long conversational sequence; in the latter case, an extended conversational sequence may be generated. It is often noted that precision is needed in order to accomplish a successful emergency intervention. Consequently, 'precision' (in locating a place') is, first, less a matter of using 'correct words' (=corresponding to an objective measuring of the world) than of using 'recognizable terms'; and, second, it is not an individual skill but rather an interactional achievement based on the organization of talk.[9]

4 Common Sense Geography

As regards the first requirement, 'giving a name of a place as a landmark' can be a sufficient resource both for callers and for call-takers to locate a place in order to respond to an emergency:

[9] On 'precision' in conversation, see Sacks (1988) and Drew (2003).

Excerpt 3.7 I Would Need the Red Cross Jeep

```
01 Caller   centodiciotto? pronto?
            one one eight? hello?
02 Ctaker   centodiciotto dica
            one one eight yes
03 Caller   ah buongiorno, rifugio vajolet
            ah good morning, vajolet refuge
04 Ctaker   sì
            yes
05 Caller   mi servirebbe la jeep della croce rossa
            I would need the red cross jeep
06          per una signora che che sta male,
            for a lady who doesn't feel well,
07          ha fatto una congestione,
            she has had a congestion,
08          non riesce più a stare in piedi
            she can't stand up anymore
09 CTaker   mh. ma posso parlare con qualcuno che l'ha vista?
            mh. but can I talk to someone who has seen her?
```

Excerpt 3.8 A Lady Who's Banged Her Head

```
01 Ctaker   centodiciotto
            one one eight
02 Caller   buongiorno abbiamo una signora
            good morning we have a lady
03          che ha picchiato la testa,
            who's banged her head,
04          siamo a san Romedio
            we're in san Romedio
05 Ctaker   a san Romedio
            in san Romedio
06 Caller   sì, e tende ad addormentarsi,
            yes, and she tends to fall sleep,
07          dove possiamo recarci al posto più vicino per::
            where is the closest place we can go in order to::
```

In Excerpt 3.7, the Vajolet refuge (line 3) is considered by the caller to be a place sufficiently familiar to be mentioned and immediately recognized in its specificity. The name of the place (in this case, a renowned refuge in the Dolomites) carries with it implicit additional information related to how to reach it. This recognizability is acknowledged by the call-taker, who provides a 'continuer' (Schegloff, 1982), (*yes*, line 4), an indicator that the call-taker has understood; that the landmark used does not need to be further specified; and that an extended unit of talk containing the reason for the call is in progress and the caller should continue (see lines 5–8).

Two requirements are at work in the sequential organization of the Excerpt 3.8. One is connected to the 'location work' by the parties; and the second is related to the activities to be accomplished next. Here the caller is not asking for assistance but for information. This kind of activity performed by the caller in his/her turn makes identification of the place less relevant to the dispatch of a first-aid vehicle and puts less pressure on the call-taker to obtain a more recognizable and identifiable location of the emergency. In fact, in this excerpt the reason for the call is in the first utterance after the greeting (another sign for the call-taker that this may not be an emergency call, as we shall see in the next chapter) (lines 2–3: *good morning we have a lady who's banged her head*); and the formulation of the place (in terms of a mutually recognizable landmark[10]) is in second position in the first caller's turn (line 4: *we're in san romedio*). In this excerpt, the understanding check (Schegloff et al., 1977) by the call-taker (line 5) invites the caller to formulate a new place reference (if the call-taker's check is taken as a lack of understanding) or to repeat the first reference (if the call-taker's check is taken as an invitation to confirm the reference). When the caller confirms the reference with a simple item (line 6, yes), then the progressivity of the call is granted with the request for information and the reference to the place is taken as understood (Schegloff, 1992).

[10] "San Romedio" is a famous Catholic sanctuary in the Trentino region of Italy.

There are many ways in which the recognizable formulation of places for organizational purposes can be achieved. There follows an example of one of the simpler cases, in which the minimal recognizable formulation of place is achieved through a formulation composed of various elements. This format shows various items connected through a 'concentric or hierarchic organization' (Schegloff, 1972), starting from the name of the city, the name of the street and the street number.[11] This is one of the standard methods of formulating a place for emergency:

Excerpt 3.9 An Ambulance Is Needed

```
01 Ctaker        centodiciotto
                 one one eight
02 C:  ah ghe    'n'emergenza qua a CITTA,
                 ah there's an emergency here in TOWN,
03               in NOME  VIA  diciasse[tte
                 seventeen ROAD NAME,
04 Ctaker        sì
                 yes
05 Caller        c'è una signora che sta male,
                 there's a lady who is ill,
06               serve 'n'ambulanza o un medico
                 an ambulance or a doctor is needed
07 Ctaker        cosa è successo? una persona che sta male?
                 what's happened? a person is ill?
```

[11] See the classification of the dispatched orders for cab drivers in Psathas and Henslin (1967, pp. 430–436). Obviously, this location description can be designed only for particular calls—that is, calls placed in a city. But emergencies happen everywhere: highways, mountains and so on, where this kind of place identification is not available. See the work of call-takers in similar, not urban situations in South Africa (Nattrass et al., 2017) and in Costa Rica (Bolaños-Carpio, 2021).

Excerpt 3.10 There Is an Emergency

01	Ctaker	centodiciotto
		one one eight
02	Caller	sì buonasera, senta c'è un'emergenza.
		yes, good evening, listen there's an emergency.
03		NOME VIA tredici a CITTA
		thirteen ROAD NAME, TOWN
04	Ctaker	sì
		yes
05	Caller	e: c'è mia suocera
		e: there's my mother in law
06		che è completamente bianca, ah
		who's gone completely white, ah
		[5 lines omitted]
12	Ctaker	ma è incosciente? è cosciente?
		but is she unconscious? is she conscious=

In both cases, the caller provides the full address (Excerpt 3.9, lines 2–3: town + name of the street + street number[12]; Excerpt 3.10, line 3: name of the street + street number + town). To be noted first is that the call-taker, once the basic formulation of the place in terms of its full address has been given, proceeds with an interrogative sequence oriented to ascertaining 'what has happened' instead of 'where it has happened' (Excerpt 3.9, line 7: *what happened?*; Excerpt 3.10, line 12: *but is she unconscious?*). This is a kind of proof procedure for the practical sufficiency and practical recognizability of place formulation between the parties. It could be said that a place formulation of a place is 'right' or adequate (for the parties) if it does not produce questions or further questions, or require reformulations (Schegloff, 1972, p. 114).[13]

[12] In Italy, the default format of an address puts the street number after the name of the street, contrary to what happens in the English-speaking countries.

[13] In the related footnote, Schegloff adds: "Right formulations need *not* be drawn from the set of "correct" formulations: it is not a set-sub-set relationship. When one office worker says to another at the end of a coffee break, 'Well, back to the salt mines', the rightness of the formulation is not precluded by the 'incorrectness' of the term as a description of his work place" (Schegloff, 1972, p. 432, footnote 15).

5 When the Geography Is Not Shared

Schegloff (1972, p. 84) notes that "the failure to report as part of the formulation of place the city's name is heard as being produced by a finding of co-presence for that formulation". This is an assumption that callers sometimes make.[14] This formulation produces an 'interactional asynchrony' between the parties as to how to recognize a place. If the formulation of town (given street and number) is missing, then shared knowledge and recognizability can be jeopardized:

Excerpt 3.11 Can You Send an Ambulance

```
01 Ctaker    centodiciotto?
             one one eight?
02 Caller    buon giorno senta
             good morning listen
03           può mandare un'autoambulanza m:: e[:
             can you send an ambulance m::: e:
04 Ctaker                                      [dove?
                                                where?
05 Caller    in NOME VIA vicino alla gelateria NAME per favore?=
             in ROAD NAME near the ice cream shop NAME please?=
06 Ctaker    =NOME VIA in che paese è? CITTA 1 o CITTA 2?
             =ROAD NAME in what town is it? TOWN 1 or TOWN 2?
07 Caller    è a CITTA[2
             it's TOWN 2
08 Ctaker             [a CITTA 2
                       in TOWN 2
09 Caller    CITTA 2 e::=
             TOWN 2 e::=
```

[14] Psathas and Henslin (1967) note that names of towns or parts of towns are "infrequently included in the order" for a cab. The town "is an element that is 'known' or understood because the dispatcher selects the cab closest to the order as the one to whom the order will be given. That selection in itself conveys the information that the order is in the same 'part of town' that the driver is in" (Psathas & Henslin, 1967, p. 432).

Excerpt 3.12 Could You Come Quickly?

```
01 Ctaker   centodiciotto?
            one one eight?
02 Caller   ah eh. podè vegnir di fat ((local dialect))
            ah eh. could you come quickly
03 Ctaker   cosa?
            what?
04 Caller   potete venire subito?
            could you come quickly?
05 Ctaker   dove?
            where?
06 Caller   eh qua in NOME VIA al numero otto
            eh here in STREET NAME number eight
07 Ctaker   in NOME VIA?
            in STREET NAME?
08 Caller   eh, al numero otto
            eh, number eight
09 Ctaker   di che paese?
            what town?
10 Caller   a CITTA 1! dove? che paese?
            TOWN 1! where? what town?
11 Ctaker   eh! qua risponde CITTA 2
            eh! here answers TOWN 2
12 Caller   e allora il centodiciotto subito per=
            and so one one eight quickly for=
13 Ctaker   =cosa è successo?
            =what has happened?
```

Excerpt 3.13 Town Missing (1)

```
01 Ctaker   centodiciotto
            one one eight
02 Caller   senta qua in NOME VIA numero sessantasei
            listen  here  in  STREET NAME number sixty six
03          dopo il NOME PIAZZA [(--)
            after  NAME SQUARE   (--)
04 Ctaker                       [qui a CITTA signo[ra?
                                 here in TOWN,  madam?
05 Caller                                         [CITTA,CITTA
                                                   TOWN, TOWN
```

Excerpt 3.14 Town Missing (2)

```
00 Ctaker    centodiciotto
             one one eight
01 Caller    sì per favore mi puoi mandare un'ambulanza=
             yes please can you send an ambulance=
02           =a NOME VIA LOCALITA
             =to ROAD NAME LOCAL PLACE
03 Ctaker    a CITTA?
             in TOWN?
04 Caller    sì a CITTA
             yes in TOWN
05 Ctaker    cosa è successo?
             what happened?
```

What should be noted in Excerpts 3.11, 3.12, 3.13 and 3.14 is that the call-taker, once a partial formulation of the place [name of the street + street number] has been given, does not go ahead with the interrogative sequence oriented to ascertaining 'what has happened'. Instead, the operators insist on getting the name of the town. Here, one element of the 'where it has happened' search is recognizably missing. When the question "*where?*" by the operator is subject to equivocality (3.12, line 5), the search for a place can be pursued by a "candidate offer" (3.11, line 6: *TOWN 1 or TOWN 2*; 3.13, line 4: *here in TOWN madam?*; 3.14, line 3: *in TOWN?*). Again, this is a kind of proof procedure for the insufficiency and unrecognizability of the place formulation between the parties. In these excerpts, the misalignment between the caller and the call-taker seems to be due to the caller's mis-assumption that the call-taker knows the location (Paoletti, 2012). The *here* (3.12, line 5) conveys a sign of immediacy and closeness to the emergency. To recall Schegloff's (1972) intuition that the participants are oriented to precision and adequacy when formulating places in talk-in-interaction, the *here* in Excerpt 3.12 can be considered the best and most elegant solution to the problem of referring to the place of a notable and momentous event. At the same time, the indexical is insufficient to the organizational reasons of the service for help.

6 When the Geography Is Shared Through Other Devices

One way for callers to be exempt from mentioning the town—and make formulation of the place recognizable—is to refer to a landmark (cf. also Bolaños-Carpio, 2021, pp. 86–88; Nattrass et al., 2017; Paoletti, 2012; Dovigo & Redaelli, 2010): that is, "a building or place that is easily recognized, especially one that you can use to judge where you are" (*Cambridge Dictionary*):

Excerpt 3.15 Castle

```
01 Ctaker   centodiciotto pronto
            one one eight hello
02 Caller   (---) dove c'è il castello NOME, in fondo, =
            (---) where the NAME castle is, at the end, =
03          =all'inizio di NOME VIA1 sì,
            =at the beginning of STREET1 NAME yes,
04          NOME VIA2, in fondo alla discesa,
            STREET2 NAME, at the bottom of the hill,
05          c'è un signore che è caduto dalla bicicletta
            there's a man who has fallen off his bike
06          e ha (---)
            and he has (---)
07 Ctaker   è cosciente? risponde 'sta persona?
            is he conscious? is this person responsive?
```

Excerpt 3.16 Health Authority Building

```
01 Ctaker   centodiciotto
            one one eight
02 Caller   buongiorno io son qua in NOME PIAZZA,
            good morning I am here in SQUARE NAME,
03          di fronte alla cassa malati,
            in front of the health authority building,
```

(*continued*)

Excerpt 3.16 (continued)

04	c'è un signore che è caduto con la bicicletta *there's a man who has fallen off his bike*
05 Ctaker	sì *yes*
06 Caller	è anche ubriaco, potete venire per favore? *he is also drunk, can you come please?*
07 Ctaker	le mando qualcuno, ma come sta adesso? *I'll send someone, but how is he now?*

Excerpt 3.17 Faculty of Economics

01 Ctaker	centodiciotto *one one eight*
02 Caller	buongiorno senta una signora *good morning listen a lady*
03	è caduta qua alla facoltà di economia *has fallen down here at the faculty of economics*
04 Ctaker	sì *yes*
05 Caller	e: (0.7) al terzo piano *e: (0.7) third floor*

These landmarks have a *metonymic relation* to the town. Mentioning a landmark in the formulation of the site of an accident does more than simply indicate a specific place: mentioning a landmark immediately 'contextualizes' the event in a broader space. The landmark is a 'part' and represents 'the whole'. Mentioning a landmark can exempt callers from mentioning large part of the area: the name of the town, the sub-region and so on, together with road, street number, access routes and so on.[15]

[15] In the domain of self-reference, Lerner and Kitzinger (2007) identify two ways of selecting terms that can be considered also for selecting place formulation: 'aggregation' or 'extraction', where the first is a change of reference from an individual to a collectivity and the second is the selection of an individual from a collectivity. Mondada (2010, p. 158) speaks of "fragmenting and reassembling heterogeneous spaces".

The extent to which this exemption is successful is part and parcel of a 'shared knowledge' and a way to show membership of a common culture. Hence, the formulation of a place through a landmark in emergency calls enables the call-takers to focus on both directions, broader and narrower, so to speak. They can 'zoom in' on the details of a territory, and 'zoom out' to the broader context at the same time. It seems the shortest and most efficient way for callers to instruct the call-takers where to send help.

Landmarks are mentioned by the callers also with a reference to the orientation of the speaker (3.15, lines 2–4: *a castle*, *at the beginning of ROAD1 NAME*, *at the bottom of the hill*; 3.16, line 3: *health authority building*, *in front of*; 3.17, lines 3, 5: *faculty of economics*, *third floor*). Thus provided is also an instructed way to read the territory in that it provides an observational point from which the scene is viewed, that is, a perspective. This way of portraying the place offers a possible disambiguating view of the landmark, which in itself may be rather vague and equivocal (in the case of the university building, which floor? In the case of a castle or a public building, where is the caller positioned?). At the same time, this description of a landmark furnishes concrete instructions regarding where to go, from which side to approach the landmark.

The name of the institution from which the call has been made, through the way in which the caller states his/her institutional affiliation, can provide the call-taker with the same multi-dimensional information about the site of the emergency:

Excerpt 3.18 Elementary School

01 Ctaker	centodiciotto *one one eight*
02 Caller	buongiorno qua è NOME SCUOLA *good morning here is the NAME OF SCHOOL*
03	CITTA quattro, = *TOWN four,=*
04	=la scuola elementare di LOCALITA *=the elementary school of LOCAL PLACE speaking*
05 Ctaker	eh con calma, non capisco *eh, calm, I don't understand*

(*continued*)

Excerpt 3.18 (continued)

```
06 Caller    sì
             yes
07 Ctaker    LOCALITA?
             LOCAL PLACE?
08 Caller    scuola elementare di LOCALITA.
             elementary school of LOCAL PLACE.
09 Ctaker    sì
             yes
10 Caller    abbiamo qua un'insegnante che non sta bene,
             we have here a teacher who doesn't feel well,
```

In this excerpt, the way in which the caller self-identifies through an institutional category is acknowledged by the call-taker (line 9) only after a repair initiator—a 'repair simpliciter' (Lerner et al., 2012; Kitzinger et al., 2013)—asking the caller to repeat his/her previous turn not because of a problem of recognition but because of difficulty in understanding (line 5).[16] The trouble here is not the reference to the place but what precedes the reference to the place, that is, a formulation that conveys information so that a specific building can be located (line 7: *LOCAL PLACE?*). The caller offers a repair to his/her previous turn by repeating the formulation (line 8: *elementary school of LOCAL PLACE*). After the simple sign of acknowledgement by the call-taker, the call continues with the formulation of the problem.

7 "Be Specific!"

We have already seen that on some occasions the search for a place initiates a sequence even before the analysis of the reason for the call, that is, the emergency problem (see Excerpts 3.11, 3.12, 3.13 and 3.14). We

[16] In Italian, "*non capisco*" ("*I don't understand*") can be ambiguous to the conversants: it can solicit a repair because the caller has either not heard well or not understood. The following turns in the sequence disambiguate the sense of this repair solicitor to the caller as a problem of hearing and not of understanding for the call-taker.

have also seen that "[p]art of the town is a dependent category in the sense that it never appears by itself". As Psathas and Henslin observe in regard to the dispatch of a cab, "A driver is not dispatched to a part of town to pick up a passenger since a large area is included within this designation. A dispatched order necessarily means that a passenger is to be located at a specific place within a part of town" (Psathas & Henslin, 1967, p. 434). Again, when this information is missing, the interrogative series from the call-taker is occupied by the work of finding a more specific place compared to what has been initially formulated by the caller:

Excerpt 3.19 Church Square

```
01 Ctaker    centodiciotto?
             one one eight?
02 Caller    sì, buongiorno,
             yes, good morning,
03           telefono da CITTA. una cosa urgente.=
             I'm calling from TOWN. urgent.
04 Ctaker    [sì
              yes
05 Caller    [=c'è una persona che si è sentita male,
              there is a person who has fainted,
06           e: è svenuta a terra.
             and: collapsed to the ground.
07 Ctaker    ma  dove? a  CITTA [dov-?
             but where? in TOWN whe-?
08 Caller                       [e::h, a CITTA,
                                 e::h, TOWN,
09           vicino a piazza della chiesa.
             near the church square
```

Excerpt 3.20 Construction Firm

```
01 Ctaker    centodiciotto
             one one eight
02 Caller    buonasera chiamo da CITTA,
             good evening I'm calling from TOWN,
03           c'è stato un incidente con una macchina
             there has been a car accident
04 Ctaker    CITTA in che via? dove?
             TOWN in what road? where?
05 Caller    sulla statale, di fronte al NOME AZIENDA,
             on the state road, in front of CONSTRUCTION FIRM NAME,
06           a nord di CITTA,
             north of TOWN,
07           prima della galleria artificiale verso i LOCALITA
             before the artificial tunnel toward LOCAL PLACE
08 Ctaker    prima (--) ah ho capito. feriti quanti?
             before (--) ah I understand. how many injured?
```

In Excerpt 3.19, after the first caller's turn in which she/he states the problem (lines 5–6: *there is a person who has fainted and collapsed to the ground*) and gives a first formulation of the place (line 3: *I'm calling from TOWN*), the call-taker asks for a specification of the place instead of continuing to ascertain the problem (line 7: *but in TOWN where?*).

In Excerpt 3.20, there is the same configuration of the sequence: just after the first caller's turn which provided a formulation of the place (line 2: *I'm calling from TOWN*), and a preliminary definition of the problem (line 3: *there has been a car accident*), the call-taker asks for a finer-grained formulation of the place (line 4: *TOWN in what road? where?*). The interrogative series about "what happened" is suspended by the call-taker until the more specific place missing from the initial formulation is stated by the caller. We shall see below how that initial request by the call-taker sets the initial step of a sequence where the caller builds a long turn which not only provides the description of the place reformulated to ensure recognition (Kitzinger et al., 2013) but also incorporates oriented instructions on how to reach the place.

8 How to Be "Specific" About Places Without Giving a Place Name

It is not rare in emergency calls that the search for place engenders a multi-turn sequence, often (but not always) put at the end of the call, before the closing sequence. The location of the accident in this case is not an elicited simple formulation of a place but amounts to an entire sequence, where the place can be identified through an incremental extension of its characteristics. See the following excerpt:

Excerpt 3.21 Door Bell

```
15 Ctaker   e il fatto che non respira bene da quanto?
            and the fact that he doesn't breathe well, since when?
16 Caller   ma  ades[so, oggi=
            but now,   today=
17 Ctaker          [ade-
                    no-
18          =oggi. va bene allora. CITTA2, via?
            =today. okay then. TOWN2, street?
19 Caller   NOME VIA- qui,
            STREET NAME- here,
20          sopra la torrefazio[ne
            above the coffee shop
21 Ctaker                      [eh qua arriva a CITTA1
                                eh here reaches TOWN1
22          signora, la telefonata,
            madam, the call,
23          mi  [deve dare via e numero
            you must give me the street and number
24 Caller       [ah! NOME VIA
                 ah! STREET NAME
25          ventiquattro
            twenty four
26 Ctaker   NOME VIA. ventiquattro?
            STREET NAME. twenty four?
```

(continued)

Excerpt 3.21 (continued)

```
27 Caller   sì
            yes
28 Ctaker   ventiquattro. COGNOME antonio?
            twenty four. FAMILY NAME antonio
29 Caller   sì
            yes
30 Ctaker   c'è  anche  COGNOME  sul  campanel[lo?
            there's also FAMILY NAME on the[doorbell?
31 Caller                                  [sì
                                            yes
32 Ctaker   okey.
            okay.
```

The sequence begins just after the call-taker has collected all the relevant information regarding the case. The end of the extended sequence devoted to collecting information on the case is marked by *okay then* (line 18), an item used to transition between a main and a subsidiary activity (Ostermann & Harjunpää, 2021; Sorjonen, 2021). The call-taker asks for the full address (line 18), which produces an initial response in the same line format as used by the call-taker (street name and number). The caller then stops and produces a place formulation through a local landmark (line 19–20: *STREET NAME, above the coffee shop*). The call-taker then asks the caller for information in the usual format of information collection about a place, which is based on street and number (line 23). At the end of this extended sequence, the call-taker takes care to collect not only the name and family name of the patient (line 28) but also assurance that this name is written on the doorbell (line 30). It seems that reaching the right place for an emergency service is connected not only to an adequate formulation of a place but also to other very practical and specific factors. Reaching the right address in terms of town, street and number and then finding a condominium with dozens of names on the intercom doorbell buzzers, where the name of the patient may not even exist, is a matter of practical difficulty for the emergency crew once it has been dispatched. The call-taker's job is to anticipate any practical problems and to ensure punctual information of localization.

This endeavour to ensure that the emergency crew reaches not only the right address but also the right person is shared by the callers. See the following excerpt:

Excerpt 3.22 Family Name

```
19 Ctaker   mi lascia il telefono e il nome della famiglia
            leave me the phone number and the family name
20 Caller   allora COGNOME,
            well FAMILY NAME,
21          sul campanello di sotto non c'è scritto niente=
            there's nothing written on the doorbell downstairs
```

The caller provides the family name when requested (line 20), but immediately adds that this would be useless information if were used to locate the patient (line 21). It seems that the caller is anticipating the possible practical difficulty of the crew dispatched in finding the right place.

The second device with which to ensure that the crew dispatched has been given enough good instructions in order to reach the place is a request for what can be called a 'transient occasional landmark' (from "transient landmark" as described by McCarthy et al., 1997, p. 07). It has been noted that there are "places with a transition value" (Schegloff, 1972, p. 101): that is, places which can be recognized not as stable final places, but as devices marking 'the way to some other place'. In particular, it is interesting that specific persons can be considered as features of places, when one person makes him/herself available to be seen in a recognizable place by the ambulance crew, so that he/she can be easily spotted. In these cases, it seems that the problem of individuation can be solved, given that the ambulance crew may reach the transient place (the place where a person would be waiting for the ambulance to arrive) from which the crew is then 'escorted' to the final destination. The place to be reached is not fixed; rather, it is variable, depending on the position in the space of this "transient landmark". This could be an essential property of coordination between caller and call-taker. See the following excerpt:

Excerpt 3.23 Send Someone into the Street

```
40 Ctaker    arriviamo subito
             we will come soon
41 Caller    sì grazie
             yes thanks
42 Ctaker    mi manda giù qualcuno in strada?
             could you send someone into the street
43 Caller    sì,    certo,
             yes, certainly,
44 Ctaker    [grazie
              thanks
45 Caller    [le mando la signora con la tenuta blu in strada.
              I'll send a lady in a blue dress.
46           va bene?
             okay?
47 Ctaker    perfetto, arrivederci
             perfect, goodbye
48 Caller    saluti grazie
             bye thanks
49 Ctaker    salve
             bye
```

In Excerpt 3.23, the call-taker reassures the caller that a crew has been dispatched and that it will soon arrive (line 40: *we will come soon*) and then asks for someone to be sent into the street (line 42). The caller answers positively (line 43), and then provides a description of the person which highlights the external characteristics useful for his/her easy identification (line 45: *a lady in a blue dress*). This is another interesting case where the description of a person is connected to the description of a place: identifying a lady with a blue dress would mean that the crew has (almost) reached the place of the emergency.

9 "But Approximately, Where Is …"

It has been pointed out (Ikeya, 2003) that the "where are you?" request in emergency phone calls does not lead to a "how to get there?" formulation. In order for ambulance crews to reach the right place, it is sometimes necessary that the caller provides a series of steps from a starting point to the destination, describing the movements through space[17]: in these cases, the callers are rendered accountable for producing a more extensive description of the place to which they are referring.

The problem of identifying "*where* something has happened" can be less banal than what appears at first sight. Even in a city, where the location of places can be made recognizable through formulation of the name of the town, address and street number, there may be problems in recognizing places: "many houses do not display a number clearly, some using a name instead; house numbers may not run consecutively: there may be clashes in street names, the same name in many different towns in the region and even the same street name used a number of times within the city" (McCarthy et al., 1997, p. 104). This is even more apparent when we move from an urban area to a mountain or country one.[18]

We have seen that localization work is mainly done through 'official' and formal definitions of places, whereas in the cases of interest to us here it is accomplished through a work of relational positioning of the main reference with other reference points in the field (see McHoul & Watson, 1984). We could argue for the existence of two kinds of knowledge: cartographic knowledge and a 'common sense geography'. The display and formulation of both is what the parties need in order to get to a recognizable location.[19]

As we have already mentioned, it often happens in emergency calls that the call-taker, after having granted the help requested by the caller, goes back in the last part of the call to the issue of the 'search for a place'. After the call-taker has collected all the relevant information, she/he resumes

[17] Relevant here are the studies by George Psathas (1979, 1986a, 1986b, 1987, 1991) on wayfinding. Cf. Liberman (2012, 2013). At the same time, the work of Psathas (and Liberman) concerns how instructions are followed. Here, the point is the way in which the caller instructs the call-taker regarding the route to follow. See also De Stefani (2018).

[18] McCarthy et al. (1997), when comparing two dissimilar areas where an emergency service is deployed—the first one serves a small predominantly dispersed, rural population and the other a large predominantly urban population—observe that "in the former, the control staff can often avail themselves of the fact that for any given area most individuals are known to each other and key individuals such as priests and publicans can be expected to know where many individuals live. In the latter, such social structures are less complete and cannot be drawn on to the same extent" (McCarthy et al., 1997, p. 109).

[19] This amounts to saying that, for instance, the region of Trentino could be described as located "between 10°30′ and 11°50′ longitude East and between 45°40′ e 46°30′ latitude North", on the one hand, or "in the North-East of Italy, near to the border with Austria", on the other. In general, on these themes see Schutz (1970), Ryle (1966), Elliot (1974) and Scott (1998).

the interrogative series, focusing again on the identification of places. These are instances in which there is much more reliance on the use of physical and geographical cues and landmarks, such as public or commonly recognizable buildings, so that call-taker and callers elaborate and verify the initial description of the place, and on concrete instructions on how to find the way. In this second case, an extended conversational sequence may be generated. See the following excerpt:

Excerpt 3.24 Approximately Where

```
37 Ctaker    e:: pressapoco dov'è di PAESE?
             e:: approximately where in TOWN?
38 Caller    prego?
             scuse me?
39 Ctaker    pressappoco dove si trova l'abitazione?
             approximately where's the house?
40 Caller    dove c'è la SUPERMERCATO
             where the SUPERMARKET is
41 Ctaker    sì
             yes
42 Caller    girate a sinistra
             turn left
43 Ctaker    SUPERMERCATO, a sinistra sì
             SUPERMARKET, left yes
44 Caller    il primo, la prima: come si dice
             the first, the first: how do you say
45           la prima viottola sempre a sinistra
             the first lane to the left
46 Ctaker    viottola a sinistra, sì=
             lane to the left, yes=
47 Caller    =andate avanti per cinquecento metri
             =go ahead for five hundred metres
48 Ctaker    sì
             yes,
49 Caller    ecco e trovate lì insomma
             right and you're practically there
50 Ctaker    va bene. okey mandiamo qualcuno allora
             okay. okay we'll send someone then
```

In this excerpt, we see the call-taker, after having secured the requested help, restarts a sequence related to the location of the emergency. His turn (line 37: *approximately where in TOWN*) projects a possible multi-turn answer, where the caller is asked to provide an extensive description of the place. The description proves to be a description of route finding. The caller, after having requested a repair (line 38), starts to give directions. He commences with a well-known point in the town (line 40: *where the SUPERMARKET is*), and then provides a sequential particular specifying the route to take: *turn left* (line 42), *the first lane to the left* (line 45), *go ahead for five hundred metres* (line 47) and then *you'll be there* (line 49). The instructions are punctuated by the call-taker's acknowledgements. He indicates an understanding of the instruction provided at each node of the journey, inviting the caller to go ahead in giving route instructions.[20] The final confirmation by the call-taker (line 50: *okay*) is followed by repetition that the help has been granted. The final confirmation of understanding is also the conversational device for signalling the conclusion of the direction-giving. Finding the place by following the instructions in situ will be the practical task of the crew mobilized for this emergency.

10 Conclusions

In this chapter, we have seen that for the call-taker to establish where an emergency has happened requires more than simply logging an address in the electronic information system, as already discussed in many papers (Frankel, 1989; Heath & Luff, 2000; Houtkoop et al., 2005; Mondada, 2010, 2011a, 2011b; Nattrass et al., 2017; Whalen, 1995a, 1995b). The computerized form has organizational requirements that account for institutional demands, and it is not designed for practical purposes (Garfinkel, 1967; Watson, 1986).

I said that we can characterize the work of formulating a place with the Gestalt metaphor of "extracting an animal from the foliage" (Garfinkel, 2022, pp. 118–119). The task of the caller in an emergency call is to render visible and recognizable, through his/her talk, the animal in the

[20] "[…] the direction-giver and direction-recipient make a great many assumptions about each other's knowledge and must continuously monitor each other's understandings. Especially, to ascertain what can be made an objective landmark the one directing must come to know the recipient's familiarity with the local area and whether what the director is providing is comprehensible to the recipient" (Liberman, 2012, p. 256).

foliage. This chapter has described some of the features of this interactional work by the caller and the call-taker. In particular, it has examined, on the one hand, the interplay of the uses of 'formal' and 'commonsense' methods in displaying knowledge of places which give rise to the recognizability of places by the call-takers and callers and, on the other hand, the sequential work of finding 'the right place'.

We have seen in this chapter how this locational work can develop in multi-turn sequences. We saw in Chap. 1 that the first turns of the callers to an emergency number contain items concerning the reason for the call. We have seen that to be found in this first turn is a characterization of the problem (the 'what') and a description of the place where the problem has occurred ('where'). Apparent in both the characterization of the trouble and the description of the place by the caller is what has been called the "preference of minimization" (Sacks & Schegloff, 1979) or "maxim of minimization" (Levinson, 1998). That is to say, due to emergency circumstances, the informative aspect of the call must be provided with minimal communicative resources—preference for minimized reference. But at the same time, there is a mandatory requirement that the characterization of the trouble and a description of the place be recognizable by the call-taker, the recipient of the emergency call—that is, under the principle of recipient design (Sacks et al., 1974),[21] there is a preference for callers to use "a reference form that will allow the recipient to recognize that a mutually known referent is being referred to"—a more general preference for intersubjectivity and common ground.

Here, there are two interactional demands in opposition: one is the 'preference for minimization'; the second is the exigency of having an accurate description of places. The progressivity of the call is impinged by the insertion sequence (often multi-turn) devoted to securing the reference to a place. But "absolute security of reference is incompatible with progressivity" (Heritage, 2007, p. 261). I suggest that progressivity of the emergency call in these cases—that is, granting help or assistance *just after* the production of the request for help or assistance (i.e., the completion of the pair "request for help—granting the request" with the actual granting of the request, in favour of the *progressivity of the action*)—is subordinated to a higher-level organization of the interaction based on the activity

[21] "By 'recipient design' we refer to respects in which the talk by a party in a conversation is constructed in ways which display an orientation and sensitivity to the particular other(s) who are the co-participants" (Sacks et al., 1974, p. 727).

(Levinson, 1992) carried out by the parties, that is, providing assistance or help (*activity progressivity*). One type of progressivity (action progressivity) is suspended in favour of another (activity progressivity), which is of a higher level (Lee, 2011). The help required cannot be provided unless the two cardinal elements for providing help—what has happened, and the precise location of the emergency—are defined and secured *for all practical purposes.*

References

Arminen, I. (2006). Social functions of location in mobile telephony. *Personal and Ubiquitous Computers, 10*, 319–323.

Bolaños-Carpio, A. (2021). Place formulation in an emergency: The case of 911 calls in Costa Rica. *Language & Communication, 80*, 80–94.

Chapman, S., & Schofield, W. N. (1998). Lifesavers and samaritans: Emergency use of cellular (mobile) phones in Australia. *Accident Analysis & Prevention, 30*(6), 815–819.

Crabtree, A., O'Neill, J., Tolmie, P., Castellani, S., Colombino, T., & Grasso, A. (2006). The practical indispensability of articulation work to immediate and remote help-giving. In *CSCW '06: Proceedings of the 2006 20th anniversary conference on Computer supported cooperative work* November, 219–228. https://doi.org/10.1145/1180875.1180910

De Stefani, E. (2018). Formulating direction: Navigational instructions in driving lessons. *International Journal of Applied Linguistics, 28*(2), 283–303.

Dovigo, F., & Redaelli, I. (2010). Knowledge management in locating the patient in an emergency medical service in Italy. *Computer Supported Cooperative Work (CSCW), 19*(5), 457–481.

Drew, P. (2003). Precision and exaggeration in interaction. *American Sociological Review, 68*(6), 917–938.

Elliot, H. C. (1974). Similarities and differences between science and common science. In R. Turner (Ed.), *Ethnomethodology. Selected readings* (pp. 21–26). Penguin.

Eriksson, M. (2010). Conceptions of emergency calls: Emergency communication in an age of mobile communication and prevalence of anxiety. *Journal of Contingencies and Crisis Management, 18*(3), 165–174.

Frankel, R. M. (1989). "I wz wondering—uhm could Raid uhm effect the brain permanently d'y know?": Some observations on the intersection of speaking and writing in calls to a poison control center. *Western Journal of Speech Communication, 53*, 195–226.

Garfinkel, H. (1967). *Studies in ethnomethodology*. Prentice-Hall.

Garfinkel, H. (2022). *Harold Garfinkel: Studies of work in the sciences* (M. Lynch, Ed.). Routledge.

Greco, L. (2004). Descriptions, catégories et collections de catégories. Le rôle de l'urgence dans le pratiques de catégorisation de la douleur dans les appels au 115. *Rivista di psicolinguistica applicate, 4*(2–3), 1–15.

Haddington, P., & Keisanen, T. (2009). Location, mobility and the body as resources in selecting a route. *Pragmatics, 41*(10), 1938–1961.

Hayashi, M., Raymond, G., & Sidnell, J. (2013). Conversational repair and human understanding: An introduction. In M. Hayashi, G. Raymond, & J. Sidnell (Eds.), *Conversational repair and human understanding* (pp. 1–30). Cambridge University Press.

Heath, C., & Luff, P. (2000). *Technology in action*. Cambridge University Press.

Heritage, J. (2007). Intersubjectivity and progressivity in person (and place) reference. In T. Stivers & N. J. Enfield (Eds.), *Person reference in interaction: Linguistic, cultural, and social perspectives* (pp. 255–280). Cambridge University Press.

Houtkoop, H., Jansen, F., & Walstock, A. (2005). Collaborative problem description in help desk calls. In C. Baker, M. Emmison, & A. Firth (Eds.), *Calling for help: Language and social interaction in telephone helplines* (pp. 63–90). John Benjamins.

Ikeya, N. (2003). Practical management of mobility: The case of the emergency medical system. *Environment and Planning A, 35*(9), 1547–1564.

Kameo, N., & Whalen, J. (2015). Organizing documents: Standard forms, person production and organizational action. *Qualitative Sociology, 38*(2), 205–229.

Kazemi, A. (2020). Fine-tuning locational formulations in mobile phone calls. *Discourse Studies, 22*(5), 553–570.

Kent, A., & Antaki, C. (2020). Police call-takers' first substantive question projects the outcome of the call. *Applied Linguistics, 41*(5), 640–661.

Kevoe-Feldman, H. (2019). Inside the emergency service call-center: Reviewing thirty years of language and social interaction research. *Research on Language and Social Interaction, 52*(3), 227–240.

Kitzinger, C., Lerner, G. H., Zinken, J., Wilkinson, S., Kevoe-Feldman, H., & Ellis, S. (2013). Reformulating place. *Journal of Pragmatics, 55*, 43–50.

Landgren, J., & Nulden, U. (2007). A study of emergency response work: Patterns of mobile phone interaction. In *Proceedings of the SIGCHI conference on Human factors in computing systems*, April, 1323–1332.

Laurier, E. (2001). Why people say where they are during mobile phone calls. *Environment and Planning D: Society and Space, 19*(4), 485–504.

Lee, S. H. (2011). Responding at a higher level: Activity progressivity in calls for service. *Journal of Pragmatics, 43*(3), 904–917.

Lerner, G. H., & Kitzinger, C. (2007). Extraction and aggregation in the repair of individual and collective self-reference. *Discourse Studies, 9*(4), 526–557.

Lerner, G. H., Bolden, G. B., Hepburn, A., & Mandelbaum, J. (2012). Granularity recalibration repairs: Refining formulations for the task at hand. *Research on Language and Social Interaction, 45*(2), 191–212.

Levinson, S. C. (1992). Activity types and language. In P. Drew & J. Heritage (Eds.), *Talk at work: Interaction in institutional settings* (pp. 66–100). Cambridge University Press.

Levinson, S. C. (1998). Minimization and conversational inference. In A. Kasher (Ed.), *Pragmatics: Vol. 4 Presupposition, implicature and indirect speech acts* (pp. 545–612). Routledge.

Liberman, K. (2012). The intelligibility of directions: The Psathas corpus. In H. Nasu & F. Chaput Waksler (Eds.), *Interaction and everyday life: Phenomenological and ethnomethodological essays in honor of George Psathas* (pp. 251–260). Lexington Books.

Liberman, K. (2013). Following sketched maps. In K. Liberman (Ed.), *More studies in ethnomethodology* (pp. 45–82). SUNY Press.

Ludwig, T., Reuter, C., & Pipek, V. (2013). What you see is what I need: Mobile reporting practices in emergencies. In *ECSCW 2013: Proceedings of the 13th European Conference on Computer Supported Cooperative Work, 21–25 September 2013, Paphos, Cyprus* (pp. 181–206). Springer.

McCarthy, J. C., Wright, P. C., Healey, P., Dearden, A., & Harrison, M. D. (1997). Locating the scene: The particular and the general in contexts for ambulance control. In *Proceedings of the international ACM SIGGROUP conference on supporting group work: The integration challenge* (pp. 101–110). Phoenix, Arizona, United States.

McHoul, A. W., & Watson, D. R. (1984). Two axes for the analysis of 'commonsense' and 'formal' geographical knowledge in classroom talk. *British Journal of Sociology of Education, 5*(3), 281–302.

Mondada, L. (2010). Reassembling fragmented geographies. In M. Büscher, J. Urry, & K. Witchger (Eds.), *Mobile methods* (pp. 138–163). New York.

Mondada, L. (2011a). Géographies mobiles et divergentes. L'établissement interactionnel des lieux d'intervention dans des appels au secours. *Revue d'anthropologie des connaissances, 5*(2), 390–436.

Mondada, L. (2011b). The management of knowledge discrepancies and of epistemic changes in institutional interactions. In T. Stivers, L. Mondada, & J. Steensig (Eds.), *The morality of knowledge in conversation* (pp. 27–57). Cambridge University Press.

Nattrass, R., Watermeyer, J., Robson, C., & Penn, C. (2017). Local expertise and landmarks in place reformulations during emergency medical calls. *Journal of Pragmatics, 120*, 73–87.

Normark, M., & Randall, D. (2005). Local expertise at an emergency call centre. In *ECSCW 2005* (pp. 347–366). Springer.

Ostermann, A. C., & Harjunpää, K. (2021). OKAY in health helpline calls in Brazilian Portuguese: Managing alignment and progressivity. In E. Betz, A. Deppermann, L. Mondada, & M. L. Sorjonen (Eds.), *OKAY across languages: Toward a comparative approach to its use in talk-in-interaction* (pp. 263–293). John Benjamins.

Paoletti, I. (2012). The issue of conversationally constituted context and localization problems in emergency calls. *Text & Talk, 32*(2), 191–210.

Pettersson, M. (2001). Talk and visibility: 'One person is out of the car—Did you hear that?'. In S. Björnestad, E. R. Moe, I. A. Mörch, & A. L. Opdahl (Eds.), *Proceedings of the IRIS 24. 11th–14th of August, 2001*, Ulvik, Hardanger, Norway, Iris. 3: 187–200. Retrieved from http://urn.kb.se/resolve?urn=urn:nbn:se:bth-9691

Pomerantz, A., & Heritage, J. (2013). Preference. In J. Sidnell & T. Stivers (Eds.), *The handbook of conversation analysis* (pp. 210–229). Wiley-Blackwell.

Psathas, G. (1979). Organizational features of direction maps. In G. Psaths (Ed.), *Everyday language: Studies in ethnomethodology* (pp. 203–226). Irvington Publishers.

Psathas, G. (1986a). Some sequential structures in direction-giving. *Human Studies, 9*(2), 231–246.

Psathas, G. (1986b). The organization of directions in interaction. *Word, 37*(1–2), 83–91.

Psathas, G. (1987). Finding a place by following directions: A phenomenology of pedestrian and driver wayfinding. *Man-Environment Systems, 17*, 99–103.

Psathas, G. (1991). The structure of direction-giving in interaction. In D. Boden & D. Zimmerman (Eds.), *Talk and social structure* (pp. 195–216). Polity Press.

Psathas, G., & Henslin, J. M. (1967). Dispatched orders and the cab driver: A study of locating activities. *Social Problems, 14*(4), 424–443.

Relieu, M. (2002). Ouvrir la boîte noire. Identification et localisation dans les conversations mobiles. *Réseaux, 112/113*(2), 20–47.

Rollet, N. (2013). "D'accord": approche conversationnelle et multimodale d'une forme située dans les appels au Samu-Centre 15. *L'Information grammaticale, 139*, 35–43.

Rollet, N. (2015). Conversations dans l'urgence. *Multitudes, 60*(3), 87–93.

Ryle, G. (1966) The world of science and the everyday world. In Id. *Dilemmas* (pp. 68–81). Cambridge University Press.

Sacks, H. (1988). On members' measurement systems. *Research on Language and Social Interaction, 22*(1–4), 45–60.

Sacks, H., & Schegloff, E. A. (1979). Two preferences in the organization of reference to persons in conversation and their interaction. In G. Psathas (Ed.), *Everyday language: Studies in ethnomethodology* (pp. 15–21). Irvington Publishers.

Sacks, H., Schegloff, E. A., & Jefferson, G. (1974). A simplest systematics for the organization of turn-taking for conversation. *Language, 50*, 696–735.

Schegloff, E. A. (1972). Notes on a conversational practice: Formulating place. In D. N. Sudnow (Ed.), *Studies in social interaction* (pp. 75–119). Free Press.

Schegloff, E. A. (1982). Discourse as an interactional achievement: Some uses of "uh huh" and other things that come between sentences. In D. Tannen (Ed.), *Georgetown University roundtable on language and linguistics: Analyzing discourse: Text and talk* (pp. 71–93). Georgetown University Press.

Schegloff, E. A. (1992). Repair after next turn: The last structurally provided defence of intersubjectivity in conversation. *American Journal of Sociology, 97*(5), 1295–1345.

Schegloff, E. A., Jefferson, G., & Sacks, H. (1977). The preference for self-correction in the organization of repair in conversation. *Language, 53*(2), 361–382.

Schutz, A. (1970). *Reflections on the problem of relevance*. Yale University Press.

Scott, J. C. (1998). Thin simplifications and practical knowledge: Metis. In Id., *Seeing like a state* (pp. 309–341). Yale University Press.

Sorjonen, M.-L. (2021). OKAY in closings and transitions. In E. Betz, A. Deppermann, L. Mondada, & M.-L. Sorjonen (Eds.), *OKAY across languages: Toward a comparative approach to its use in talk-in-interaction* (pp. 94–127). John Benjamins.

ten Have, P. (2002). The notion of member is the heart of the matter: On the role of membership knowledge in ethnomethodological inquiry. *Forum Qualitative Sozialforschung / Forum: Qualitative Social Research, 3*(3). https://doi.org/10.17169/fqs-3.3.834

Watson, D. R. (1986). Doing the organizations work: An examination of a crisis intervention centre. In S. Fisher & A. D. Todd (Eds.), *Discourse and institutional authority* (pp. 91–120). Ablex.

Whalen, J. (1995a). Expert systems versus systems for experts: Computer-aided dispatch in public safety communication. In P. Thomas (Ed.), *The social and interactional dimensions of human-computer interfaces* (pp. 161–183). Cambridge University Press.

Whalen, J. (1995b). A technology of order production: Computer-aided dispatch in public safety communication. In P. ten Have & G. Psathas (Eds.), *Situated order. Studies in the social organization of talk and embodied activities* (pp. 187–230). University Press of America.

Whalen, M. R., & Zimmerman, D. H. (1987). Sequential and institutional contexts in calls for help. *Social Psychology Quarterly, 50*(2), 172–185.

Zimmerman, D. H. (1992a). Achieving context: Openings in emergency calls. In G. Watson & R. M. Seiler (Eds.), *Text in context: Contributions to ethnomethodology* (pp. 35–51). Sage.

Zimmerman, D. H. (1992b). The interactional organization of calls for emergency assistance. In P. Drew & J. Heritage (Eds.), *Talk at work: Social interaction in institutional settings* (pp. 418–469). Cambridge University Press.

Zimmerman, D. H. (1998). Identity, context and interaction. In C. Antaki & S. Widdicombe (Eds.), *Identities in talk* (pp. 87–106). Sage.

CHAPTER 4

When a Call Is Not an Emergency

Abstract This chapter deals with calls that are not emergency calls. In particular, I examine how callers design their turn so that the call-taker immediately realizes that the call is not an emergency. I show that formulating the action one is doing is a powerful method to make clear what the speaker is doing. I analyse cases in which the caller uses a formulation to make it clear that she/he is asking for information, not asking for help.

Keywords Non-emergency calls • Formulations • Information requests • Entitlements and contingencies

Calls arriving at an emergency call centre are particularly interesting for those who study communication, for several reasons. Here, 'effective communication' is certainly not a slogan from managerial training courses; rather, it is a practical necessity, with major consequences on the state of affairs in the world (where sometimes people's very lives are at stake). Operators need to know with good approximation ('for all practical purposes', Garfinkel would say) 'what has happened' and 'where it has happened' to make the best use of the rescue apparatuses at their disposal. Having 'good information' is the result of the assiduous interactional work in which emergency call centre operators are constantly engaged. As a rule, this interactional work of seeking and assembling relevant information is done under time pressure: there is no time for a complete

G. Fele, *Emergency Communication*,
https://doi.org/10.1007/978-3-031-26239-5_4

reconstruction of the facts (which requires the most precise and timely information to be acquired), while it is necessary to act as rapidly as possible. A first sense of the word 'emergency' lies in this constraint to provide an adequate response to the call for help as quickly as possible—and this constraint may be at odds with the need to thoroughly investigate the nature and origin of the problem at hand.[1] A second sense of the word 'emergency' refers to the fact that events that require the provision of help are not planned—nor are they plannable (Petterson and Rouchy, 2002). Although there is a wide range of expectations that orient the attention of dispatchers, it is common to hear call-takers say that "each case is distinct", "each event is singular", "each call is unique", "every time it's like starting from scratch", and so on.[2] Call-takers are prepared for typical scenarios for typical places (e.g., an emergency call made from a construction site is likely to be about a work accident and a call from the highway is likely to be about a road accident). Or, they may be prepared for situations that typically occur at certain times of the year, in certain months, weeks and even hours of the day, or ones related to the weather (Raymond & Zimmerman, 2007). In a mountain area, at weekends in winter, more calls are expected for traumas on ski slopes; when it rains, there may be motorcycle accidents; and so on. Yet it is never known in advance when exactly an event needing the provision of help may occur. A call for emergency intervention may be made during the day, at night, in the afternoon, in the early morning, on New Year's Eve, on Sunday and Monday and so on; there may be long moments of 'calm'; two or even more events may occur at the same time or in rapid succession; and so on. To some extent, one might say that workers in an operations centre 'expect the unexpected'.

For all these reasons, the work of emergency operators is of particular interest to those involved in communication. A social researcher who considers the phone calls made to an operations centre is faced with a dense and rich body of material in which many 'things' happen in the span of

[1] As Booker et al. (2018, p. 13) say, "There will always be a conflict between the caller's agenda of receiving a resolution *as quickly as possible*, and the institutional agenda of providing a resolution *as quickly as necessary*."

[2] Wennlund et al. (2022) identify with "being creative in gathering information" and "continuously processing and assessing complex information", two basic qualities attributed by the operators in emergency medical communication centres in Sweden to their work.

sometimes only a few seconds. The caller's very first turn-at-talk is of capital importance for the call-taker to start to gain an understanding of the ongoing events and orient the following sequences of talk.

1 Asking for Information

Consider these three excerpts of calls received by the 118 operations centre:

Excerpt 4.1 Splinters of Wood

```
01 Ctaker    centodiciotto?
             one one eight
02 Caller    sì buongio- buon giorno, scusi,
             yes good- good morning, sorry,
03       →   posso: chiederle un'informazione?
             can: may I ask you for some information?
04 Ctaker    per cosa?
             regarding what?
05 Caller    eh eh c'ho un bambino piccolino
             eh eh, I have a very young child
06           che ca- cadendo praticamente
             who fal- falling practically
07           si è appoggiato con le mani,
             put his hands down,
08           era- eravamo sa in un rifugio
             we we-, we were you know in a refuge
09           qua: in provincia di Trento
             here: in the province of Trentino
10           sa, e: si è infilato nel- nella manina
             you know, a:nd he got in- in his little hand
11           delle scheggette di legno.
             some splinters of wood.
```

Excerpt 4.2 Intestinal Flu

```
01 Ctaker   centodiciotto
            one one eight
02 Caller   sì buongiorno, senta,
            yes good morning, listen,
03   →      volevo un'informazione innanzitutto.
            I want some information above all.
04          se è possibile.
            if it's possible.
05 Ctaker   mi dica
            tell me
06 Caller   eh senta, noi siamo a PAESE,
            eh listen, we are in VILLAGE
07          NOME   frazione, no?
            NAME OF THE locality, right?
08 Ctaker   sì
            yes
09 Caller   mio papà è un cardiopatico,
            my father is cardiopathic
10          fatto sta che ieri pomeriggio:
            the fact is that yesterday afternoo:n
11          gli è venuta un'influenza intestinale
            he got intestinal flu
```

Excerpt 4.3 Renal Colic

```
01   (bip)
02 Ctaker   pronto? (.) pronto?
            hello? (.) hello?
03 Caller   pronto?
            hello?
04 Ctaker   pronto:. buonasera mi dica,
            hello:, good evening tell me,
05          centodiciotto Trento.
            one one eight Trento.
```

(continued)

Excerpt 4.3 (continued)

```
06 Caller→    eh buonasera senta, vorrei un'informazione.
              eh good evening listen, I need some information.
07            una ragazza che ha delle convulsioni=
              a girl with convulsions=
08 Ctaker     =sì
              yes
09 Caller     ha un principio di colica renale,
              has started to have renal colic,
10            può fare una puntura di Buscopan?
              can she have an injection of Buscopan?
```

These are three phone calls (taken from a group of other similar cases) about events that are not treated as emergencies by the caller. The chapter starts precisely with this question: How can a call be made to an emergency number in such a way that it embodies and exhibits that the case 'is not an emergency?'. What pattern does the caller's turn exhibit? What kind of interactional work do the parties (both the caller and the call-taker) do so that they can reach a shared 'definition of the situation'?

The cases under consideration would seem to be ones in which the callers are engaged in making the situation clear to their interlocutor, beyond any possible misunderstanding, at the very first opportunity to do so. The work of making the situation as clear as possible by the callers for the call-takers—beyond all possible ambiguities in action ascription (Stivers et al., 2022)—is required all the more because the communicative situation is oriented towards the application of a certain kind of interpretive frame to the actions of the participants ("here we respond to emergency requests"). Orletti (1983) explains that making explicit the kind of action that someone is doing is an instruction to the addressee regarding how a turn should be considered, minimizing possible misunderstanding in order to achieve a shared reading of the situation. It is a way to anticipate any action ascription: that is, the interpreting work of Ego that is responsive to prior turns of Other (Deppermann & Haugh, 2022). Drew (2022) describes how participants work to avoid or disguise particular action ascriptions. In the cases that I have presented, we witness the opposite kind of work by the participants: in the very first turn, the caller's work is that of making as clear as possible to the call-taker what she/he is doing in his/her turn. In certain particular situations, this way of explicitly *naming* the kind of action that one is doing is the focal point of the interaction. It is one of the few cases in social interaction where one participant says in so many words what she/he means, what she/he intends to say, directly. Garfinkel and Sacks (1970, p. 171) called turns of this kind "formulations": that is, forms of meta-communication practice by which the conversationalists explicitly describe what they are doing: "What they are doing is saying-in-so-many words-what we-are-doing."[3] One of the examples that Garfinkel and Sacks give of formulations is when a conversationalist explains and describes what she/he is saying. And formulations are powerful devices to make clear what a participant is saying: "Formulations are a principal means participants use to display and secure that their interactions are self-explicative, intelligible and accountable events" (Deppermann, 2011, p. 117). Orletti provides some concrete examples: "the complex of formulation practices is used by conversationalists from time to time to define what is being done (e.g., 'We are discussing between friends, not arguing'), who is speaking, and the characteristics of the interactants (e.g., 'You are speaking to your boss'), at what point one is in the development of the discourse (e.g., 'To conclude…'), what one or the other of the conversationalists 'really' said (e.g., 'I wanted to say that'), in which place someone is (e.g., 'Children, we are in the house of strangers'), what one is talking about or will talk about (e.g., 'Today we will deal with the problem'), whose turn it is to speak (e.g., 'I was speaking'), etc." (Orletti, 1983, p. 85).

In conversation analysis, there is now an extensive body of literature concerning the use and functions of 'formulations', the expressions that explicitly describe what is being done when something is said (see Deppermann, 2011). Paul Drew (2003) has described the use and function of formulations in various institutional contexts. For example, in psychotherapy sessions, patients may use formulations to clarify the meaning and implication of an overtly vague observation by the therapist. In radio programmes that involve telephone calls from a home audience, formulations may be used by the programme's host to construct a particular, tendentious version of what the person who is intervening in the broadcast has said, triggering a sequence of disagreement or confrontation. In television news interview programmes, formulations are used by journalists to prompt

[3] For an earlier treatment of formulations, see Heritage and Watson (1979, 1980). More recently, see Deppermann (2011) and Van der Houwen and Sliedrecht (2016).

or encourage the interviewee to provide new details on the subject, often trying to enliven the interview. In industrial negotiations between unions and management, one side may offer a formulation of what the other side is proposing in order to build a compromise which the other side can accept, thus closing a phase regarding the subject of the dispute. Some crucial aspects of formulations concern the form in which they can be constructed (interrogatively or declaratively, for example), the lexical choices they involve and the prosodic and sequential aspects of their construction.

Most of these studies have considered formulations as second actions: that is, the ways in which a receiver exhibits his/her reading and interpretation of a previous turn. In the cases that I have presented, the formulations appear instead in the very first turn of the caller to an emergency number; they are Ego's and not Other's concern.

A characteristic of this first turn of the callers is that the formulation engenders a sequence. Consequently, we have to consider the meta-communicative aspect in its sequential placement (Orletti, 1983, pp. 87–91—see also Heritage & Watson, 1979, 1980). This means not simply finding a 'home for orphans' (Goffman, 1981, p. 30), i.e., placing expressions that in themselves would be fully intelligible in a 'context', but thoroughly explaining the work that these expressions do at the moment they are used (according to the "why that now" motto of conversation analysts). With these considerations in mind, I return to the cases presented earlier.

2 Formulations and Their Sequential Context

Telephone conversations are interesting, from an analytical point of view, because the communicative resources available to the participants involve only the oral-aural channel, to the exclusion of sight (Svensson and Hällgren, 2018). This makes in particular the initiation of telephone conversations even more interesting because, basically, people have to introduce themselves 'verbally' reciprocally and precisely within the space of a few lines, in fleeting moments. We have seen how this is an important aspect of emergency calls. We have also seen that in 'ordinary' phone calls there is generally a certain preliminary routine that allows the caller to open a conversation and to arrive step by step at the reason for the call, whereas in phone calls to emergency centres everything happens much more rapidly. Typically, in emergency calls, the second turn of the call (the first for the caller) is occupied immediately by the presentation of the problem and the request for help.

This is the context of emergency communication: the ringing of the call opens a horizon of expectation in the operations centre that is immediately 'filled with meaning' by the caller as soon as the channel is available and she/he has evidence that the service has been reached. The caller's problem is this: How can an action that is not an emergency request (such as asking for information) be carried out in such specialized context in a way that leaves no room for doubt or does not produce misunderstanding?

One possible solution is precisely the production of a formulation in this context. With a formulation, the caller makes explicit, makes manifest and makes immediately transparent the kind of action that she/he is taking. What is interesting is that the caller at that point, in his/her first turn-at-talk, does not take the opportunity to ask straightforwardly for information. This option may still foreshadow an emergency. The caller replaces the act of asking for information with a formulation that says, "I am making a request for information".

This is what happens in the three excerpts presented above. In different grammatical forms (Excerpt 4.1, line 3: *can I ask you for information?*; Excerpt 4.2, line 3: *I want some information, if possible*; Excerpt 4.3, line 6: *I need some information*), the callers use a formulation to make explicit the kind of action that they are doing at that moment. The formulation thus performs a fundamental disambiguating function in the talk: by formulating that an item of information is needed. Instead of going ahead with the request for information, the formulation makes clear that what is being requested is not the dispatch of help. It is a way to clarify that the call is not for an ambulance but for an item of information.

Let us also look at the composition of the caller's entire turn, the one that contains the formulation. It is apparent that the formulation is accompanied by other elements that 'water down' the emergency potential of the caller's turn. The formulation does not appear immediately. Nor is the caller's turn occupied only by the formulation; it contains elements preliminary to the formulation, such as the following: items acknowledging the call-taker's summons (Excerpt 4.1, line 2: *yes*; Excerpt 4.2, line 2: *yes*; Excerpt 4.3, line 6: *eh*); greetings (Excerpt 4.1, line 2: *good morning*; Excerpt 4.2, line 2: *good morning*; Excerpt 4.3, line 6: *good evening*); various types of tokens (Excerpt 4.1, line 2: *sorry*; Excerpt 4.2, lines 2 and 6: *listen*; Excerpt 4.3, line 6: *listen*). All these elements exhibit marked and non-preferred traits. In contrast, the call to action for an emergency is made up of unmarked turns that contain preferred elements.

Hence, in the first place the formulation has a *retrospective* function: it indexes an explicit response to the previous action (that of the dispatcher, who answers to the summon with "one one eight"), orienting the interpretation of the caller's current action and the expectations of the call-taker in that sequential context. But of course, this formulation has an important *prospective* function: it refers to a series of actions to come that are now promised and announced (Goodwin, 1995). As Garfinkel and Sacks (1970, p. 176) said, "doing formulating is not the definitive means whereby the fact is itself done or established. The question of what one who is doing formulating is doing [...] is not solved by members by consulting what the formulation proposes, but by engaging in practices that make up the essentially contexted character of the action of formulating." That is to say, the formulation used by the caller is 'tested' and checked in the subsequent development of the call: that the call really implies that no request for intervention is reviewed at each following turn of the conversation.

The sequential perspective is broadened at this point: it is no longer about the fact that a formulation opens a pair of adjacent elements that has to be closed by a second pair part; rather, it concerns the prefiguration of an extended sequence to come. In all three excerpts, the call-taker effectively closes the pair of adjacent elements:

Excerpt 4.4 Splinters of Wood, Lines 08 and 09—from Excerpt 3.1

```
03 Caller→   posso: chiederle un'informazione?
             can: may I ask you for some information?
04 Ctaker    per cosa?
             regarding what?
```

Excerpt 4.5 Intestinal Flu, Lines 05, 06 and 07 from Excerpt 4.2

```
03 Caller→   volevo un'informazione innanzitutto.
             I want some information above all.
04           se è possibile.
             if it's possible.
05 Ctaker    mi dica
             tell me
```

Excerpt 4.6 Renal Colic, Lines 15, 16 and 17—from Excerpt 4.3

```
06 Caller→    eh buonasera senta, vorrei un'informazione.
              eh good evening listen, I need some information.
07            una ragazza che ha delle convulsioni=
              a girl with convulsions=
08 Ctaker     =sì
              yes
```

I would point out that the closure of the pair of adjacent elements by the call-taker takes the form not so much of an acceptance or rejection of the formulation as of authorization or denial of the action presaged by the caller's formulation. In all three cases, the call-taker authorizes continuation of the interaction in the manner presaged by the formulation. Thus, the formulation projects a long sequence, of which it constitutes only a 'preliminary' (Terasaki, 1976). A typical feature of a sequence of this kind is that the turn following the authorization is not immediately occupied by the action prefigured in the formulation (a question by which the request for information is made), but by a series of elements preliminary to the re-request itself: this is, as Schegloff well observed (Schegloff, 1980), a case of 'pre-pre.' See the following excerpt:

Excerpt 4.7 Renal colic, Lines from 15 to 19 from Excerpt 4.3

```
06 Caller→    eh buonasera senta, vorrei un'informazione.
              eh good evening listen, I need some information.
07            una ragazza che ha delle convulsioni=
              a girl with convulsions=
08 Ctaker     =sì
               yes
09 Caller     ha un principio di colica renale,
              has started to have renal colic,
10            può fare una puntura di Buscopan?
              can she have an injection of Buscopan?
```

The caller's formulation (line 6: *I need some information*) is not followed by the actual question, but by an extended turn consisting of three macro-elements, only the last of which is the question proper. The macro-elements (line 7: *a girl with convulsions*; line 9: *has started to have a renal colic*) are composed of contextual information that prepares the question (line 10: *can she have an injection of Buscopan?*). Thus, the caller's initial formulation functions as a preliminary to a preliminary: the formulation is placed before the contextual background, which in turn is placed before the actual information request.

Above (Excerpt 4.4 and Excerpt 4.5), I have only partially reported the sequence, which occupies several turns. Now, in the following, I can show the extended excerpt:

Excerpt 4.8 First Aid Station

30	Caller	fatto sta (oggi), le dicevo,
		the fact is (today), I was telling you,
31		che io ho chiamato la guardia medica
		that I called the first aid station
32	Ctaker	┌sì
		yes
33	Caller	└a CITTA', no?=
		in TOWN, right?=
34	Ctaker	=sì
		=yes
35	Caller	però, eh:: continua::,
		but, eh:: it keeps-
36		c'è la segreteria telefonica.
		there is the answering machine.
37		ho lasciato il mio messaggio ma non-,
		I left my message but I don't-
38		si vede che è fuori, non so.
		it looks like he is out, I don't know.
39	Ctaker	mh mh mh=
40	Caller	=ma voi potete darmi
		=but can you give me
41		il numero del cellulare del dottore?
		the doctor's cell phone number?

The actual request for information (lines 40–41: *but can you give me the doctor's cell phone number*?) is formulated by the caller after a long preparation made by producing contextual elements (regarding the difficulty of contacting the first aid station, which is also a way to show to the call-taker that the call to the emergency number has been made only after other options have been tried).

In Excerpt no. 4.9, the production of contextual elements means that the operator can anticipate the caller's formulation of an explicit question. The operator can thus 'provide an answer' (lines 33–34: *I can give you the number of the tourist medical service*) even without an actual question fully formulated by the caller:

Excerpt 4.9 First Aid Station for Tourists

```
29 Ctaker     mah, se vuole, le posso dare
              well, if you want it, I can give you
30            il numero della guardia medico tur-,
              the number of the first aid station for tour-
31            della: (eh, sì), siete turisti voi?
              of (eh, yes), are you tourists?
32 Caller     sì, sia┌mo turisti
              yes, we are tourists
33 Ctaker→           └le posso dare
                      I can give you
34    →       il numero della guardia medica ┌turistica,
              the number of the first aid station for tourists
35 Caller                                    └sì
                                              yes
```

To a large extent, from a sequential point of view, the function of initial formulation by the callers (Excerpt 4.4, line 3: *may I ask you for some information*?; Excerpt 4.5, lines 3–4: *I want some information, if possible*; Excerpt 4.6, line 6: *I would like some information*) is to secure a longer following turn-at-talk. It is in this way that the problem can be fully described by the caller. Hence, the formulation is a solution to the problem of finding a negotiated and shared definition for the progressivity of the interaction.

Let us conduct a thought experiment concerning calls in which callers immediately request the information that they need. Consider the case of Excerpt 4.5, where the caller, immediately after the call-taker's response (*one one eight?*), asks, *can you give me the cell phone number of doctor XY?*. Or, consider the case in Excerpt 4.6: *can a girl who has convulsions and the onset of renal colic have an injection of Buscopan?*. One might reasonably expect such an action to engender a 'suspicious' reaction in the call-taker, who seeks to ascertain what kind of emergency intervention might be required. "Why do you need the doctor's number? But how is the girl now?" It is not that operators are 'suspicious' by nature: it is the organization itself of interaction and conversation that structures systems of expectations. Initial formulations by callers channel the meaning of an action so that its meaning is immediately recognized.

3 Entitlement and Contingency

In a study on an emergency dispatch system in Costa Rica, Bolaños-Carpio (2020) observed that whereas in life-threatening incidents or ones of severe urgency callers tend to request help via a description, in the case of non-life-threatening incidents or ones of limited urgency they tend to request help in a more cautious manner, often using the phrase "*para ver si*" ("to see if"). Referring to the work of Curl and Drew (2008), Bolaños-Carpio (2020) noted that callers in their turns (via grammar and turn design) display an entitlement to making a request (i.e., the speaker's right to ask for something) and an orientation to the contingencies connected with fulfilling the requested action. In life-threatening situations, it usually happens that the caller designs his/her turn so that she/he can claim high entitlement and a strong right to make a request, exhibiting scant acknowledgement of contextual factors that might impede the realization of his/her request, as we have seen in Chap. 1. When the caller's turn exhibits a claim of low entitlement and a weak right to make a request, exhibiting strong acknowledgement of the contextual factors conditioning realization of his/her request, the call-taker is instructed that the call is probably not—for the time being, in that particular moment in the sequence—about a non-life-threatening case.

If we return to the excerpts presented above, we see how the turns were designed in those cases: Excerpt 4.4, line 3: *may I ask you for some information?*; Excerpt 4.5, lines 3–4: *I want some information, if possible*; Excerpt 4.6, line 6: *I would like some information*. In all the cases, it seems that the turn construction conveys the caller's low entitlement and his/her high considerations of the contingencies that may impede fulfilment of the request. It seems that the callers orient "to the possibility that the assistance might not be provided (i.e, it is a high contingency request) and, possibly, to [...] low entitlement to the request" (Bolaños-Carpio, 2020, p. 244).

See also the following excerpt:

Excerpt 4.10 A Package Like That of a Cake

```
01 Ctaker    polizia?
             police?
02           (.)
03 Caller    pronto?
             hello?
04 Ctaker    sì è polizia, pronto
             yes, it's the police, hello
05 Caller    sì salve
             yes, hello
06 Ctaker    [(----)
07 Caller    [io sto uscendo dal parcheggio di: CITTA'
              I am leaving the car park in TOWN
08 Ctaker    sì?
             yes
09 Caller:   non so se è interessante,
             I don't know if it is interesting,
10           però è una cosa un po' sospetta
             but it's something rather suspicious
11 Ctaker    cioè?
             what?
12 Caller    cioè vicino alla:: a un bidone dell'immondizie
             that is, near to a trash can
13           c'è un pacco come quello di una torta,
             there is a package like that of a cake,
14           chiuso per bene con il suo:,
             well sealed with its,
```

(*continued*)

Excerpt 4.10 (continued)

```
15              con il [suo fiocchettino
                with its little bow,
16 Ctaker             [mh
17 Caller       appoggiato per terra.
                laid on the ground.
18 Ctaker       m.
19 Caller       io non so, io (.)
                I don't know, I (.)
20              manderei una macchina a dargli un'occhiata,
                I'd send a car to take a look at it,
21              vedete voi
                it's up to you
22 Ctaker       ma dove questo?
                 but where is it?
```

In this call to the emergency police number, the caller, after having secured being on the line with the police and having greeted the call-taker, starts to describe the place from where he is calling (line 7: *I am leaving from the car park in TOWN*). The turn is designed as the beginning of a story, not as the description of a problem. From the outset, this place description conveys a sort of casual, not intentional looking, bringing to some unplanned encounter during his normal activity in everyday life (not the result of a continuous paranoid search for sources of danger). The place is described in transitory terms, indicating that the caller was not spending time there purposedly. After the positive response from the call-taker (line 8: *yes*) acknowledging the previous turn and granting continuation of the account, the caller does not continue a story but hedges it with a statement that does not commit him too deeply (lines 9–10: *I don't know if it is interesting, but it's something rather suspicious*). With this hedging, the caller manifests his low entitlement to any request to follow—the caller's turn seems to be completely oriented to the contingencies that can impede fulfilment of the request. The caller demonstrates his concern but at the same time is willing to rely on the call-taker's expertise in deciding whether or not the matter reported has to be considered a problem warranting action. After the call-taker's request to specify the problem, the caller finally describes it in lines 12–17: *near to a trash can there is a package like that of a cake, well-sealed with its little bow, laid on the ground.* The description provided by the caller implies that he has encountered some inconsistencies and explains why he has called the police: it seems to be a rather innocuous package, except for the fact that it is well sealed (not unwrapped, as when a package has been opened to see its contents), near to a trash can (usually, near to trash cans there are opened packs with their contents ready to be treated as garbage, not as food), and lying on the ground (sealed packages should be in more appropriate places, like on tables, not on the ground).

Usually, in a call to an emergency number, the description of the problem is followed by a response from the call-taker, who can proceed in the interrogation series. In this case, the call-taker produces a minimal acknowledgement token (line 18: “m”) that invites the caller to continue. It is at this point that the caller produces his turn with an open request for an intervention: *I don’t know, I’d send a car to take a look at it, it’s up to you* (lines 19–21). The way in which this request is formulated shows the low entitlement of the caller and a recognition of the plausible circumstances in which the emergency service could be that would make the request hard to fulfil. Showing signs of uncertainty (*I don’t know*), and characterizing his observation as made from a lay perspective, in contrast to that of a professional agent, the caller shapes his turn as a friendly suggestion (Couper-Kuhlen, 2014, p. 635) made by a non-qualified person, rather than a solid request with reasonable grounds. And again, the suggestion places the onus of the decision on the call-taker.[4]

4 Conclusions

We have seen how the activity of requesting help can be modulated by the caller. There are substantial grounds to argue that callers’ first turns that exhibit dispreferred features—not presenting at the first opportunity the problem for which help is sought; inserting greetings and other time-consuming tokens; providing personal names in a context where usually no personal names are given—embody a non-urgent reason for calling. In these cases, the call-taker is instructed to expect some sort of minor urgency. The callers may be oriented to the fact that asking for help has costs, and that the service is provided only if the reasons for doing so are well grounded and robust. In the ways in which they design their turns, in

[4] On how callers discursively construct risk through categories which enable them to make sense of the dangers they perceive, see Rock (2018).

the ways in which they display entitlement to ask for help and recruit assistance, callers embody the right and prerogative to request succour. At the same time, callers are oriented towards the contingencies that call-takers may encounter in dispatching aid. We have also seen that one of the ways in which callers exhibit their orientation towards the constraints and demands of the emergency response system is the formulation of the action in which she/he is engaged in the very first turn, making the non-emergency nature of the call explicit. It is interesting to note that the usual way in which a caller communicates a sense of emergency, when there is one, is not to formulate it at the very beginning ("this is an emergency"), since it would be considered an unnecessary waste of time in the process of recruiting assistance (even if it could be found later in the call to issue a complaint against the call-taker when the interrogation series is perceived an obstacle to having an immediate and fast response).

In any case, the significance of the call and the status of the emergency are made evident in the sequential unfolding of the call, during the interrogation series, confirming the caller's orientation and formulation of the problem, but also sometimes recasting it as a more serious matter warranting the deployment of assistance and the dispatch of urgently needed aid.

References

Bolaños-Carpio, A. (2020). When emergencies are not urgent: Requesting help in calls to the 9-1-1 Costa Rica. In C. Taleghani-Nikazm, E. Betz, & P. Golato (Eds.), *Mobilizing others: Grammar and lexis within larger activities* (pp. 229–252). John Benjamins Publishing Company.

Booker, M. J., Shaw, A. R., Purdy, S., & Barnes, R. (2018). 'Primary care sensitive' situations that result in an ambulance attendance: A conversation analytic study of UK emergency '999' call recordings. *BMJ Open, 8*(11), e023727.

Couper-Kuhlen, E. (2014). What does grammar tell us about action? *Pragmatics, 24*(3), 623–647.

Curl, T. S., & Drew, P. (2008). Contingency and action: A comparison of two forms of requesting. *Research on Language and Social Interaction, 41*(2), 129–153.

Deppermann, A. (2011). The study of formulations as key to an interactional semantics. *Human Studies, 34*(2), 115–128.

Deppermann, A., & Haugh, M. (Eds.). (2022). *Action ascription in interaction*. Cambridge University Press.

Drew, P. (2003). Comparative analysis of talk-in-interaction in different institutional settings: A sketch. In P. Glenn, C. LeBaron, & J. Mandelbaum (Eds.), *Studies in language and social interaction: In honor of Robert Hopper* (pp. 293–308). Lawrence Erlbaum.

Drew, P. (2022). The micro-politics of social actions. In A. Deppermann & M. Haugh (Eds.), *Action ascription in social interaction* (pp. 57–82). Cambridge University Press.

Garfinkel, H., & Sacks, H. (1970). On formal structures of practical actions. In C. Mckinney & E. A. Tiryakian (Eds.), *Theoretical sociology* (pp. 338–366). Appleton Crofts.

Goffman, E. (1981). *Forms of talk*. University of Pennsylvania Press.

Goodwin, M. H. (1995). Assembling a response: Setting and collaboratively constructed work talk. In P. ten Have & G. Psathas (Eds.), *Situated order: Studies in the social organization of talk and embodied activities* (pp. 173–186). University Press of America.

Heritage, J., & Watson, D. (1979). Formulations as conversational objects. In G. Psathas (Ed.), *Everyday language: Studies in ethnomethodology* (pp. 123–162). Irvington.

Heritage, J., & Watson, D. (1980). Aspects of the properties of formulations in natural conversations: Some instances analysed. *Semiotica, 30*(3–4), 245–262.

Orletti, F. (1983). Pratiche di glossa. In F. Orletti (Ed.), *Comunicare nella vita quotidiana* (pp. 77–103). Il Mulino.

Raymond, G., & Zimmerman, D. H. (2007). Rights and responsibilities in calls for help: The case of the Mountain Glade Fire. *Research on Language and Social Interaction, 40*(1), 33–61.

Rock, F. (2018). 'Apparently the chap is a bit of a rogue': Upgrading risk in non-emergency telephone calls to the police. *Journal of Applied Linguistics and Professional Practice, 13*(1-3), 276–301.

Schegloff, E. A. (1980). Preliminaries to preliminaries: 'Can I ask you a question?'. *Sociological Inquiry, 50*(3–4), 104–152.

Stivers, T., Rossi, G., & Chalfoun, A. (2022). Ambiguities in action ascription. *Social Forces*. soac021. https://doi.org/10.1093/sf/soac021

Svensson, M., & Hällgren, M. (2018). Sensemaking in sensory deprived settings: The role of non-verbal auditory cues for emergency assessment. *European Management Journal, 36*(3), 306–318.

Terasaki, A. (1976). Pre-announcement sequences in conversation. In G. Lerner (Ed.), *Conversation analysis: Studies from the first generation* (pp. 171–223). John Benjamins.

Van der Houwen, F., & Sliedrecht, K. Y. (2016). The form and function of formulations: Co-constructing narratives in institutional settings. *Journal of Pragmatics, 105*, 55–58.

Wennlund, T. K., Kurland, L., Olanders, K., Khoshegir, A., Kamil, H. A., Castrén, M., & Bohm, K. (2022). Emergency medical dispatchers' experiences of managing emergency calls: A qualitative interview study. *BMJ Open, 12*(4), e059803.

CHAPTER 5

How to Ask for Help When There Is Little or No Information

Abstract This chapter deals with a possible problem in calling for help. Often the call is made by a third person who has limited or no knowledge of what has generated the need for an emergency intervention. Claims by the caller of limited or no knowledge about the case are delicate interactional matters because the caller should be able to offer grounds for his/her request. I show the ways in which callers deal with this problematic aspect in their turns, and the conditions under which help is nevertheless granted even in the absence of information.

Keywords "I don't know" • Insufficient knowledge • Knowledge and responsibility • Calls on behalf of a third party

1 Knowledge and Responsibility in Emergency Calls

It is assumed that a caller to an emergency number is in a privileged position with regard to the event that has taken place and requires some type of emergency intervention. This close proximity to the event enables the caller to provide important information that may be required by the call-taker. This chapter deals with cases in which the caller lacks the

G. Fele, *Emergency Communication*,
https://doi.org/10.1007/978-3-031-26239-5_5

information required for assistance following an emergency call.[1] We have already examined the call-taker's task of collecting information and the ways in which the caller responds to questions asked by the call-taker (Whalen & Zimmerman, 1987, 1990; Whalen et al., 1988; Zimmerman, 1984, 1992a); but a substantial number of emergency calls are made when the caller has limited knowledge or no knowledge at all of the circumstances of the incident. This lack of knowledge is often due to the fact that the caller is not directly involved in, or has not been a direct witness to, the event, but is merely someone who has been delegated by someone else to make the call (Tennent, 2021). As previous studies have shown, operators do not consider a simple request for an emergency service to be a reason for providing it unless some additional communicative work is done to collect basic information about what has happened, and when. Through a series of questions put to the caller, call-takers attempt to obtain the best possible information about the nature of the event and the place where it has occurred. The particular purpose of this series of questions is to ascertain the reliability and accuracy of the information provided by the caller. In other words, the description that the caller produces (regarding the nature of the event, what has happened, and where, etc.) must enable the service to assess the genuineness of the problem and the appropriateness of the request (Whalen & Zimmerman, 1990; Heritage & Clayman, 2010).

This chapter focuses on what happens in emergency calls when a caller cannot provide the essential information regarding the event for which she/he is asking for help: for example, information on what has happened and where. Knowledge of facts about the event is crucial for the delivery of the service by the emergency organization. In order to be authoritative, and therefore to receive the attention and the service required as rapidly as possible, the caller must be a credible witness to the event; and she/he should possibly have first-hand knowledge of what has happened. But what happens when the caller has no knowledge, or only second- or even third-hand knowledge of what has happened, and is not an eyewitness to the event?

I have selected for this chapter a smaller corpus of calls where instances of qualified stand-alone 'I don't knows' appear in the conversations.

[1] Mondada (2011) provides a detailed analysis of a conference call in a call centre dealing with the problem of locating a caller searching for help, in which the participants' lack of knowledge is indexed by epistemic verbs in their negative form (as *je ne sais pas*, *je ne connais pas*, *je ne vois pas* in French).

2 How the Display of a Lack of Knowledge Can Have the Consequence of the Request for Help Being Rejected

I start with analysis of 'not knowing claims' by considering their position in various sequential environments of the call for help. First, I argue that a 'no knowledge claim' can seriously impinge on the progressivity (Stivers & Robinson, 2006) of the call. If a 'no knowledge claim' is made during the very first steps of the set of questions after a request for help has been made (e.g., for an ambulance), the caller is seen as lacking the necessary grounds for making the request.[2] In these cases, if the caller is unable to account for his or her request, then the progressivity of the entire activity will be impaired: that is, the call will soon be brought to a close and the service will not be provided.[3] Let us consider the first excerpt:

Excerpt 5.1 I Got a Call from Her Mother

```
01 Ctaker    centodiciotto
             one one eight
02 Caller    eh buongiorno som e::l NOME COGNOME,
             uh, good morning. my name is NAME FAMILY NAME
03           LOCALITA. g'ho bisogn dell'ambulanza.
             LOCAL PLACE. I need an ambulance
      ...
((5 lines omitted))
      ...
09 Ctaker    cosa è successo?
             what's happened?
10 Caller    non lo so, m'ha telefonà so mama,
             I don't know, I got a call from her mother,
11           (------) (l'è venù for), (----)
             ((incomprehensible)) (it has come out), ((incompr.))
```

(*continued*)

[2] Booker et al. (2018) highlight how challenging it can be to triage calls when the problem is 'unknown' to the caller.

[3] On the police officers' rejection of requests of intervention in call to a duty desk of an Oslo police station, see Rønneberg and Svennevig (2010).

Excerpt 5.1 (continued)

```
12            (guarda) la m'ha dit, dì de ciamarghe l'ambulanza,
              (look) she told me, tell him to call the ambulance
13            perché mi non- ↓hh↓ ↑hh↑ ((sospiri))
              because I can't ↓hh↓ ↑hh↑ ((heavy breathing))
14 Ctaker     allora, facciamo una cosa, lei ha la possibilità
              well, let's do this, do you have the chance
15            di farmi chiamare:,
              to have someone else call me
          ((the call continues))
```

Here we witness the serious implications of 'not knowing claims' for continuation of the overall sequence and a (positive) conclusion of the activity. The telephone call begins with a request for an ambulance (line 3: *I need an ambulance*) without a reason for the request being provided. We have seen in previous chapters and from the work of Zimmermann (1984, 1992b) that 'interrogative sequences' are produced by emergency operators to ascertain the basis of a request for help, to decide whether the reasons provided by the caller meet the organization's criteria and to provide a definitive response to the initial request (for which the preferred answer is granting the service required). Given the lack of relevant information about the case in the caller's very first statement, the operator begins the interrogation (line 9: *what's happened?*). In terms of conversational organization, the interrogation series is a kind of "pre-second insert expansion" (Schegloff, 2007, pp. 106–109): that is, "preliminary to some particular type of second pair part which has been made relevant next by the type of first pair part to which it is responding [...] pre-second inserts look forward, ostensibly to establish the resources necessary to implement the second pair part which is pending". The caller's response to the operator's request for information contains the "claim of insufficient knowledge" *I don't know* (line 10). This claim is followed by a kind of account of the reason for this lack of knowledge, which is ostensibly obscure (line 10–13). Given both the claim of insufficient knowledge and the opaque reason for the request, the operator does not proceed with the interrogation series, but turns back to the focus of the call—a request for help—and asks the caller to find another, more knowledgeable, person who can make a second call (line 14–15: *Let's do this, do you have the chance to have someone call me?*). The initial request for help is thus turned down. The call-taker's turn shows the non-preferred nature of the action of not granting the request (Vinkhuyzen & Szymanski, 2005; Rønneberg & Svennevig, 2010; Lee, 2011b).[4]

Contrary to what has been shown to happen in ordinary conversation (Stivers & Robinson, 2006), in the above excerpt the insufficient knowledge claim is produced without delay or a preface: it is produced in the first position of the turn. In this way, the caller is shown to be willing to answer the operator's question. While this may be considered sufficient for the purposes of promoting the progress of the sequence type so far (giving the answer to a question), it is not enough to proceed with the interrogation series in order to continue the activity (providing help or service). The insufficient knowledge claim (together with an opaque reason for the lack of information) turns the interaction back to the high-order organization of the call (Lee, 2011b), presaging closure of the activity.

It can be said that in this case the entitlement to ask for an ambulance displayed by the caller is high, given the form in which the request is made (line 3, *I need an ambulance*) (Drew & Walker, 2010; Curl & Drew, 2008). At the same time, the caller fails to provide the high level of entitlement to what is requested with a robust grounding in regard to the specific details of the case.

3 How an Insufficient Knowledge Claim May Be Associated with a Strong Entitlement

I now turn to a second point. We have seen that if the 'not knowing claim' is delivered by the caller in the very first slot, where the caller is asked to provide information about the case at hand (in this way he or she will show entitlement to make a request), then the request is deemed to be groundless, and the risk that it will be turned down is at its highest. Conversely, if the 'not knowing claim' is made by the caller before the call-taker has asked any questions regarding the incident, the caller is seen as providing sufficient entitlement to make the request, especially if some kind of reason for the caller's lack of knowledge is also provided. In these cases, the call normally proceeds with the interrogation series (which is usually oriented to ascertaining where the problem has happened, not what has happened). See the following excerpt:

[4] Lee (2011a) examines how agents in commercial service encounters design their conduct when customers' requests cannot be granted.

Excerpt 5.2 A Lady Who Saw Him Told Me to Call

```
01 Ctaker   centodiciotto pronto::?
            one one eight
02 Caller   buonasera è caduto uno un-,
            good evening. someone has had a fall
03          uno con un (------)
            someone with a (------)
04 Ctaker   dove?=
            where?=
05 Caller   =a Vano,
            =in Vano,
06          a Rigo Vano
            Rigo Vano
07 Ctaker   cioè, a Rigolo Vano?
            that is, Rigolo Vano?
08 Caller   sì, pe- la strada per Bomberano.
            yes, along the road to Bomberano.
09          (.)
10          (senta), mi ha detto una signora che l'ha visto di:,
            (listen), a lady who saw him told me to
11          di chiamare,
            to call,
12          quindi io non so nie[nte
            so I don't know anything
13 Ctaker                       [ma lei non sa niente?
                                 but you don't know anything?
14          non ha visto: che:
            you didn't see what:
15          che problemi ha, né niente?
            what kind of problem he has, or anything?
16 Caller   niente=
            nothing=
17 Ctaker   =ma eh dove si trova a Rigo Vano?
            =but, uh, where are you in Rigo Vano?
```

As in the first excerpt, the insufficient knowledge claim (*I don't know*) appears during the initial stages of the call (line 12). Unlike in the first excerpt, however, the call does not begin with an overt request for an ambulance but with a report of a problem (it is not fully audible in the audio, but a paraglider has crashed to the ground—lines 2–3). This manner of presenting a problem is a strong form of entitlement: the depiction of the situation (even one as undeveloped as that seen in this excerpt) demonstrates a strong claim on the part of the caller that the situation is sufficiently severe to warrant an intervention without it being necessary to make an explicit request for one.

The call-taker then turns to the interrogative series, and asks for the location of the accident, which is then developed and identified by the parties (lines 4–7). Just after confirmation by the caller of the correct name of the place (the place names have been replaced with pseudonyms), a short gap in the conversation occurs. The caller has just provided the information required by the operator, but the call-taker has not yet granted the intervention that has been sought. This short gap presages possible difficulty in granting the intervention: the second pending part of the 'report of an accident/provision of assistance' pair is missing. In particular, the gap could be interpreted as projecting the call-taker's scepticism about the events depicted by the caller. It is at this point that the caller starts talking again: *listen, a lady who saw him told me to call, so I don't know anything* (lines 10–12). First, in the reason that he gives for his call (*a lady who saw him told me to call*), the caller places responsibility for the seriousness or accuracy of the information provided (Raymond & Zimmerman, 2007, p. 35) on the shoulders of another person, while at the same time reaffirming his duty to report the fact after being requested to do so (see also below in Sect. 5.3). Second, by 'claiming no knowledge' so powerfully (Keevallik, 2011) (*so I don't know anything*, line 12), he is saying that the situation is a consequence of his position with regard to the event; it has not arisen because he has initiated a demanding action without having the necessary entitlement to do so, or before he has acquired the requisite information. In this way, the caller anticipates the potentially negative outcome of his call: that is, having his request for help turned down. He shows that he is willing to answer the operator's question, while at the same time his position with respect to the events is marked as lacking important information.

We have seen in Excerpt 5.1 that one of the ways in which a call-taker can turn down a request is to ask to the caller to find another, more knowledgeable, person to make a second call. In this case, there seems to be no such resource, because the caller *is* the person whom someone has asked to call. *He* already is this second person. Reporting the case as it is, is the way in which the caller-as-reporter can show his relationship to the event and demonstrate how 'thin' his knowledge of the situation is, due to his position in relation to it. This 'thin', or 'skinny', reporting is subsequently packaged as indirect reported speech (lines10–11: *a lady [...] told me to call*), marking an interesting shift in evidentiality: the caller is characterizing his description as a second-hand, or reportative, experience, while at the same time characterizing the origin of the information as a knowledgeable person, to whom direct evidentiality is given because it derives from the first-hand sensory experience of the original person (*a lady* who saw him *told me to call*).

The call-taker addresses the caller's state of no knowledge by verifying the amount of knowledge that he can show (lines 13–15: *but you don't know anything? you didn't see what kind of problem he has, or anything?*). After receiving confirmation that the caller has no knowledge at all about the case (line 16: *nothing*), the call-taker goes ahead with the interrogation series and asks for more information about the location of the caller in the place from where he is calling (line 17: *but, uh, where are you in Rigo Vano?*). When the caller first reveals his state of no knowledge about the event for which he is asking for help, even in an aggravated manner, accompanied by the statement that his is a 'reported report', he is seen to be entitled to make the request. While this may not be sufficient for gathering more information about the case (which is a prerequisite for accepting or refusing the request), it is enough to recognize the right of the caller to make the request and promote the progress of the interrogation series so as to go ahead with the activity (providing help or the service). The claim of insufficient knowledge that the caller self-produces (together with a well-grounded and reasonable explanation for the lack of information) permits a return to the high-order organization of the call (Lee, 2011b), thereby preventing the early closure of the activity.

4 How the Display of Lack of Knowledge Can Have Only Local Consequences in the Interaction

We have seen that in calls for help the caller is required to be able to show that he or she has knowledge of the event for which help is being requested, whereas the call-taker is in a situation in which she/he knows nothing about it (this is a case of "absolute epistemic disadvantage"; see Heritage, 2013, p. 377). The two excerpts considered so far illustrate cases in which the caller's display of lack of knowledge about the event is interactionally managed in different ways, and with a different outcome: in the first case, the sending of help is not granted[5], while in the second case it is not compromised. In terms of management of the conversation, a demonstration of no or limited knowledge about the case for which the caller is asking for help has potentially serious consequences for the progressivity of the call: if the caller has no information, the information-seeking interrogation series cannot continue; the caller is seen as not being entitled to make a request, and the call may be brought to a close, presaging the fact that the request for help will not be granted.

There are cases in which the caller has some knowledge about the event, but only a limited amount; the caller is able to provide a general picture of the problem, or the unfortunate event, but is not able to provide full details. The call-taker's task is to ascertain whether the limited knowledge of the caller is sufficient or insufficient grounds for organizational and institutional purposes. Again, a failure to provide any information may impact on the progressivity of the call; and the likelihood that the request for help will be turned down is higher.

We have seen (in Excerpt 5.2) that when 'no knowledge claims' are made by the caller, they may be accompanied by reasons and motives. The caller is oriented towards being cooperative with the call-taker in that he or she marks the insufficient knowledge as due to the limited positioning or partial access to the scene, and not as due to declining the responsibility to respond. In these cases, the call is expected to go ahead, often with a change of topic, and the progressivity of the activity and the granting of help can be saved. Let us now look at Excerpt 5.3:

[5] For an analysis of a call arrived in a Japanese emergency call centre regarding an incident with fatal consequences after an ambulance request was rejected, see Hayashi (2019).

Excerpt 5.3 There's Been an Accident

01	Ctaker	centodiciotto?
		one one eight
02	Caller	signora, sono sull'autostrada e da Trento
		madam, I'm on the motorway from Trento
03		(stiamo andando) verso Modena.
		(we're heading) towards Modena.
04		c'è stato un incidente.
		there's been an accident.
05	Ctaker	ma dove?
		but where?
06	Caller	eh, siamo a Trento,
		eh, we are in Trento,
07		siamo subito dopo Trento, siamo.
		we are immediately after Trento, we are.
08	Ctaker	ma, in direzione sud, comunque?
		but, southbound, anyway?
09	Caller	in direzione sud, sì.
		southbound, yes.
10	Ctaker	eh, ma eh, quante macchine-, cioè,
		uh, but uh, how many cars-, that is,
11		quanti feriti ci sono.
		how many injured people are there?
12	Caller	eh, uno grave, penso, signora.
		uh, one severely, I think, madam.
13	Ctaker	ma è cosciente, risponde, parla?
		but is he conscious, does he respond, is he talking?
14	Caller	non lo so, guardi,
		I don't know, you see,
15		perché io l'ho appena visto.
		because I've only just seen him.
16	Ctaker	signora, il chilometro dell'autostrada,
		madam, the kilometre number of the motorway,
17		me lo può dire almeno?
		can you tell me that, at least?

In this case, a description of a problem is provided by the caller (line 4: *there's been an accident*). This description may be interpreted as a kind of indirect request for help (Whalen & Zimmerman, 1987; Heritage & Clayman, 2010) in which the caller is seen to present a problem to the service without asking for the service or claiming that the service should be provided: it is as if the caller is fully aware that the call-taker can decide how to intervene without any claim being made regarding the necessity of sending help, because the emergency is self-evident. This is a case of low contingency/high entitlement: as Drew and Walker (2010, p. 110) say, "[i]n emergency calls, [...] callers can seem to claim a great degree of entitlement, and a concomitant lower level of contingency, than may seem to be warranted by 'the facts'—or rather, their account/descriptions of the facts, circumstances, etc., of the incident."

The call-taker's response to this description, which is a question about the location of the problem (line 5: *but where?*), indicates that the event depicted merits an intervention, and the call-taker starts to seek the information necessary to send help. After gathering information about the location of the accident (lines 5–9), the call-taker turns to the accident itself, first asking for details about the cars involved and then, after self-repair, about the people who may have been involved in the accident (lines 10–11: *how many cars-, that is, how many injured people are there?*). This is the first question from the call-taker that is oriented towards obtaining more details. The caller's answer shows that her access to the state of affairs about which she has been requested to provide information is uncertain. The use of "I think" (line 12: *one severely, I think, madam*) casts the information provided about how many people have been involved in the accident and the seriousness of the injured people's condition not as a report of a straight state of affairs, but rather as a subjective evaluation signalling the speaker's uncertainty about the information required. The evidence of her description is taken from a mediated act, from an act of reflection, and not from a direct assessment or professional expertise. "I think" is one of the most common markers for doubt or uncertainty (Kärkkäinen, 2003, 2006), and in terms of epistemic status it marks the caller as giving an uncertain first-hand account of the status of an event.

The call-taker goes on to gather information about the seriousness of the injury mentioned by the caller (line 13: *but is he conscious, does he respond, is he talking?*). The way the question is formulated invites the caller to confirm or disconfirm three potential different statuses of the injured person by a simple yes/no answer. This is one of the customary ways in which a call-taker designs questions so that the caller's answer can be simplified. The form of the call-taker's question requires no statement or description from the caller about a complex set of various conditions of the injured person. It merely requires confirmation or disconfirmation of a series of features of medical interest, regarding which the caller only needs to 'check and say'. In these cases taken from emergency calls, the 'yes/no type interrogative' is a constraint for a conforming answer (Raymond, 2003) which focuses only on specific aspects of the scene; the 'yes/no type interrogative' works as an aid for the caller so that she/he can shape a response in the desired direction without losing time and relevance.

The response from the caller claims no knowledge and offers reasons and an explanation for why the information requested was not acquired (line 14: *I don't know, you see, because I've only just seen him*). The caller has characterized her first response turn about the accident more in the form of a tentative guess than as an adequate knowledgeable report describing an actual state of affairs (through the use of "I think"), but now she gives no access at all to the information requested. Again, this is a claim of no knowledge about a detail of the case. Claiming no knowledge has no consequence for the overall organization of the conversation. The caller is seen to have entitlements for making a request for help. Her state of no knowledge is justified by an unfavourable position in the field, and it is not the result of an uncooperative response to the call-taker's initiatives. The state of no knowledge regarding even an important detail of the accident does not impinge on the progressivity of the call. Just after, the call-taker offers signs of being only slightly disturbed (lines 15–16: *madam, the kilometre number of the motorway, can you tell me that, at least?*), while continuing the interrogative series.

5 How to Avoid Making Claims of Insufficient Knowledge and Have the Request for Help Considered

Finally, I analyse ways to avoid making claims of insufficient or no knowledge after a request for information has been made. Two procedures for grounding a request for help under conditions of limited or no knowledge are particularly worthy of mention. One is connected with the mitigation of the state of affairs by means of a stand-alone "I think" (or "I don't think") or "it seems so", where the description of the problem is not presented as indisputable, but only as the product of a guess or a personal opinion. We have just seen an instance of this "epistemic downgrading" (Heritage & Raymond, 2005) in Excerpt 5.3. The second procedure which I want to analyse briefly at this stage is packaging the report of the problem in indirect reported speech—placing the burden of making the request for help on a third party, and not the actual caller (this is similar to what we have seen in Excerpt 5.1). In these cases, I shall avoid an analysis based exclusively on lexical terms (such as "I don't know") (Sert & Walsh, 2013) and consider the ways in which a lack or shortage of information does not impinge on the activity under way. Let us now look at Excerpt 5.4:

Excerpt 5.4 Stung by a Bee or a Wasp

01	Ctaker	centodiciotto *one one eight*
02	Caller	centodiciotto, sì buonasera, *one one eight, yes good evening,*
03		sono dell'APT di Trento. *I am an APT employee in Trento.*
04		mi è appena stato riferito che c'è una persona *I've just been told that there is a person*
05		in piazza Dante, che è stato punto *in Piazza Dante, who's been stung*
06		da un'ape o una vespa *by a bee or a wasp*
07		ed è allergico ed inizia ad avere reazione *and he's allergic and is beginning to have a reaction*
08	Ctaker	e sta avendo la reazione? *and is he having the reaction now?*
09	Caller	così mi è stato riferito= *that's what I've been told=*
10	Ctaker	=non le han detto se è cosciente, *=didn't they tell you if he's conscious,*
11		se è incosciente= *if he's unconscious?=*
12	Caller	=al momento è ancora cosciente *=at the moment he's still conscious*

What is interesting here is how the caller responds to the first question from the call-taker, *this is what I've been told* (line 9). Let us see how the call begins. After a categorical self-presentation (line 3: *I am an APT employee in Trento*), no explicit request for help can be found in the caller's first turn. The caller presents the case warranting intervention by reporting an event that has been related to him (a person has just been stung by a bee or a wasp and is having an allergic reaction). The reported event is framed by the fact that the event is not the product of a personal experience of the caller: the caller is not a witness to the event, and he has no first-hand experience of the case he has reported. He has *just* been told about the event: in this "*just*" we see all the urgency of the matter; whether the caller has been asked to make the call to the emergency service or whether the call has been made on the caller's personal initiative is not clear at this early stage of the call.

In the presentation of this problem, we can see a shift from the reported fact to the act of reporting. In terms of entitlement to make a request, the use of indirect reported speech places the burden of responsibility on the person who actually saw the person suffering from the sting and who was able to witness the allergic reaction. The adoption of a reportive epistemological stance has the effect of making the speaker less responsible for the information. The grounds for a request may be shaken, and the sending of the help requested may depend on the capacity of the caller to add additional information to the reporting provided in the first turn. The caller will be seen as entitled to make the request if he is able to show that he possesses information about the case even though he is at least one step removed from the direct experience of the witness.

The call-taker starts the interrogation series in order to discover more about the case. She does so by repeating the last sentence of the caller's previous turn (line 8: *and is he having a reaction?*). The way in which the call-taker's turn is formulated gives the listener the opportunity to confirm the item of information provided in the first turn, or to clarify it (by adding new details). In this way, the call-taker probes the caller about his status as a reliable person in order to determine whether he can provide a strong basis for his knowledge. This is the response by the caller: *that's what I've been told* (line 9).

By answering in this way, the caller does not address the factual information that the call-taker has sought, but only the fact that the information given previously was the product of what someone other than himself had said. Not only does this freestanding *that's what I've been told* mark a "reportive epistemological stance" (Mushin, 2001)—in which knowledge of information is marked as not being part of the speaker's direct experience and the source of knowledge is another person—but the caller is also able to hide his position as a non-knowledgeable person. By not answering "I don't know" to the call-taker's question and presenting himself as a mere reporter, the caller is attempting to make the best of the situation in which he is asking for help, but he is aware that his request for help requires entitlements that he cannot give. By repeating that he is making a request on behalf of another person, the caller makes it clear that he lacks the actual grounds for a request and offers his position for assessment by the call-taker, while at the same time offering his duties and responsibilities as person who has been asked by another person to make a call and request help. Finally, he makes no commitment as to the truth, adequacy or completeness of the situation depicted in his first description of the emergency.

The call-taker probes the caller's levels of knowledge and reliability by asking for a specific detail on the presumed condition of the patient (lines 9–10: *didn't they tell you if he's conscious, if he's unconscious?*). The caller is able to continue providing information, which this time is not framed by any "reportive epistemological stance" markers (line 12: *at the moment he's conscious*). The call continues, and the likelihood that the help requested will be granted is now greater. The free-standing *that's what I've been told* has prevented any overt claim of lack of knowledge and assures the speaker sufficient entitlement to make a request even under conditions of limited or uncertain information.

6 Discussion

My starting point for this chapter has been the issue of knowledge displays in conversation and the rights and obligations in social interaction associated with knowing something. Participants in a conversation are expected to make claims regarding states of the world to which they have at least some degree of access: they are expected to 'know' what they are talking about (Grice, 1975). The second line of my discussion has dealt with requests and a speaker's entitlements concerning a request. According to Labov and Fanshel (1977), in order for a request to have solid grounds, the speaker must be heard to have the right to tell the listener to take the required action, and there must be the desire to take this action. The various ways in which requests are made in social interaction (request design) reveal various orientations on the part of the speakers regarding their entitlements or rights to make a request: the more explicit or straightforward the request, the more the speakers claim the right to have their requests granted (Curl & Drew, 2008).

In social interaction, members use subtle ways to advance their rights, and to request actions by their interlocutors based on their entitlement to do so. In some cases, requesting an interlocutor to do something can be more difficult, because the requester fails to furnish the necessary grounds for his/her request. The alleged entitlement to make a request must be commensurate with the knowledge displays of the case at hand. The empirical cases here come not from mundane interaction but from an institutional format, that is, the calls arriving at an emergency call centre. We have seen a sample of cases of calls to an emergency number, where the caller makes a request for help but is not able to provide the evidence or relevant knowledge which might confirm that he or she has the presumed entitlement. We have seen what happens when the urgency to receive a service is accompanied by a state of limited or no knowledge as the basis for issuing the request. We have seen two types of social relevance at work in opposite directions in these cases: the relevance and urgency of obtaining help, on the one hand, and the importance of having information before any offer of service will be possible on the other.

I started the analysis with instances of "I don't know" provided by a caller when asked about the case (or details of the case) for which he or she was calling for help. "I don't know" is a conversational formula used for a "claim of insufficient knowledge" (Beach & Metzger, 1997). Many studies have documented the ways in which "I don't know" is used to perform a variety of different actions in everyday conversation and various institutional contexts (see Baumgarten & House, 2010; Beach & Metzger, 1997; Diani, 2004; Drew, 1992; González-Martínez, 2008; Grant, 2010; Hutchby, 2002; Keevallik, 2011; Pichler, 2009; Scheibman, 2000; Sert & Walsh, 2013; Tsui, 1991; Weatherall, 2011). The cases of claims of insufficient knowledge that I have analysed in this chapter are qualified 'stand-alone' tokens and are mainly used in a literal sense.[6] In response to an information-seeking question, "I don't know" states an inability to provide the information requested. In emergency calls, claims of insufficient knowledge are frequently made as a response to a request for information:

[6] This chapter does not offer an analysis of cases in which a claim of insufficient knowledge is used as an alert for some type of subsequent approximation, used as a "preliminary hedging practice". See Weatherall (2011).

this answer functions as a second pair part, but does not provide the response for which the question was first put. I have analysed how claims of insufficient or absent knowledge can jeopardize the entire emergency call in the course of which a request for help is made because they are interpreted by the call-taker as indexing insufficient grounds for making the request. Claims of insufficient or no knowledge affect not only the sequence's local organization but also the activity's entire organization.

7 Conclusions

This chapter is, first, a contribution to the study of the social distribution of knowledge in social interaction, in particular of claims of 'insufficient or no knowledge claims' where a display of knowledge is requested; second, it contributes to the study of the relations between request design and a display of commensurate knowledge that makes the speaker fully entitled to make a request; and finally, it is a contribution to the study of emergency calls, with a particular focus on the relations among the terms of knowledge, the grounds for the request and provision of the requested service.

I have shown that when a display of knowledge is requested, a claim of "insufficient or no knowledge" is a delicate interactional matter: it is "a highly sensitive act and has social consequences" (Keevallik, 2011, p. 184). I have sought to show how an insufficient or no knowledge claim has different consequences if it is produced in response to a previous question or is self-provided, and whether or not it is accompanied by reasons or motives of the lack of knowledge. We have also seen ways to avoid using insufficient knowledge claims even when the speaker's access to the required information is completely lacking. The second issue relates to the ways in which this 'insufficient or no knowledge claim' is connected with entitlement to make a request. I have shown that granting a request is associated with the ability of the requesting party to demonstrate to the interlocutor that he or she has the entitlements to make such a request. Inability to show a basis and grounds for the request impinges on the chance of having the request granted. I have shown the conditions under which a request might be granted even where the knowledge on which a request should be based is lacking. Finally, I have sought to furnish additional insights into the dynamics of emergency calls, in particular by analysing how a service is provided or not provided and help is dispatched or not dispatched, given the grounds for the request, the entitlements of the caller and the information at his or her disposal.

References

Baumgarten, N., & House, J. (2010). I think and I don't know in English as lingua franca and native English discourse. *Journal of Pragmatics, 42*(5), 1184–1200.

Beach, W. A., & Metzger, T. R. (1997). Claiming insufficient knowledge. *Human Communication Research, 23*(4), 562–588.

Booker, M. J., Shaw, A. R., Purdy, S., & Barnes, R. (2018). 'Primary care sensitive' situations that result in an ambulance attendance: A conversation analytic study of UK emergency '999' call recordings. *BMJ Open, 8*(11), e023727.

Curl, T. S., & Drew, P. (2008). Contingency and action: A comparison of two forms of requesting. *Research on Language and Social Interaction, 41*(2), 129–153.

Diani, G. (2004). The discourse functions of "I don't know" in English conversation. In K. Aijmer & A. Strenström (Eds.), *Discourse patterns in spoken and written corpora* (pp. 157–171). John Benjamins.

Drew, P. (1992). Contested evidence in courtroom cross-examination: The case of a trial for rape. In P. Drew & J. Heritage (Eds.), *Talk at work* (pp. 470–520). Cambridge University Press.

Drew, P., & Walker, T. (2010). Citizen's emergency calls to police: Requesting assistance in calls to the police. In M. Coulthard & A. Johnson (Eds.), *Handbook of forensic linguistic* (pp. 95–110). Routledge.

González-Martínez, E. (2008). Des réponses "je ne sais pas" lors d'une enquête sociale. *Bulletin suisse de linguistique appliquée, 88*, 19–41.

Grant, L. E. (2010). A corpus comparison of the use of "I don't know" by British and New Zealand speakers. *Journal of Pragmatics, 42*(8), 2282–2296.

Grice, P. (1975). Logic and conversation. In P. Cole & J. Morgan (Eds.), *Syntax and semantics. Vol. 3: Speech acts* (pp. 41–58). Academic Press.

Hayashi, R. (2019). Categorization for occasioned semantics: Reanalysis of a Japanese Yamagata 119 emergency call. *Discourse Studies, 21*(5), 495–521.

Heritage, J. (2013). Epistemics in conversation. In J. Sidnell & T. Stivers (Eds.), *Handbook of conversation analysis* (pp. 659–673). Wiley-Blackwell.

Heritage, J., & Clayman, S. E. (2010). Calls for emergency service. In J. Heritage & S. Clayman (Eds.), *Talk in action: Interactions, identities, and institutions* (pp. 53–100). Wiley-Blackwell.

Heritage, J., & Raymond, G. (2005). The terms of agreement: Indexing epistemic authority and subordination in talk-in-interaction. *Social Psychology Quarterly, 68*(1), 15–38.

Hutchby, I. (2002). Resisting the incitement to talk in child counselling: Aspects of the utterance 'I don't know'. *Discourse Studies, 4*(2), 147–168.

Kärkkäinen, E. (2003). *Epistemic stance in English conversation: A description of its interactional functions, with a focus on 'I think'*. John Benjamins.

Kärkkäinen, E. (2006). Stance taking in conversation: From subjectivity to intersubjectivity. *Text and Talk, 26*(6), 699–731.

Keevallik, L. (2011). The terms of not knowing and social affiliation. In T. Stivers, L. Mondada, & J. Steensig (Eds.), *The morality of knowledge in conversation* (pp. 184–206). Cambridge University Press.

Labov, W., & Fanshel, D. (1977). *Therapeutic discourse: Psychotherapy as conversation*. Academic Press.

Lee, S. H. (2011a). Managing nongranting of customers' requests in commercial service encounters. *Research on Language and Social Interaction, 44*(2), 109–134.

Lee, S. H. (2011b). Responding at a higher level: Activity progressivity in calls for service. *Journal of Pragmatics, 43*(3), 904–917.

Mondada, L. (2011). The management of knowledge discrepancies and of epistemic changes in institutional interactions. In T. Stivers, L. Mondada, & J. Steensig (Eds.), *The morality of knowledge in conversation* (pp. 27–57). Cambridge University Press.

Mushin, I. (2001). *Evidentiality and epistemological stance. Narrative retelling*. John Benjamins.

Pichler, H. (2009). The functional and social reality of discourse variants in a northern English dialect: I Don't Know and I Don't Think compared. *Intercultural Pragmatics, 6*(4), 561–596.

Raymond, G. (2003). Grammar and social organization: Yes/no interrogatives and the structure of responding. *American Sociological Review, 68*, 939–967.

Raymond, G., & Zimmerman, D. H. (2007). Rights and responsibilities in calls for help: The case of the Mountain Glade Fire. *Research on Language and Social Interaction, 40*(1), 33–61.

Rønneberg, K., & Svennevig, J. (2010). Declining to help: Rejections in service requests to the police. *Discourse & Communication, 4*(3), 279–305.

Schegloff, E. A. (2007). *Sequence organization in interaction: A primer in conversation analysis*. Cambridge University Press.

Scheibman, J. (2000). I dunno: A usage-based account of the phonological reduction of don't in American English conversation. *Journal of Pragmatics, 32*(1), 105–124.

Sert, O., & Walsh, S. (2013). The interactional management of claims of insufficient knowledge in English language classrooms. *Language and Education, 27*(6), 542–565.

Stivers, T., & Robinson, J. D. (2006). A preference for progressivity in interaction. *Language in Society, 35*(3), 367–392.

Tennent, E. (2021). "I'm calling in regard to my son": Entitlement obligation and opportunity to seek help for others. *British Journal of Social Psychology, 60*(3), 870–887.

Tsui, A. B. (1991). The pragmatic functions of I don't know. *Text-Interdisciplinary Journal for the Study of Discourse, 11*(4), 607–622.

Vinkhuyzen, E., & Szymanski, M. H. (2005). Would you like to do it yourself? Service requests and their non-granting responses. In K. Richards & P. Seedhouse (Eds.), *Applying conversation analysis* (pp. 91–106). Palgrave Macmillan.

Weatherall, A. (2011). I don't know as a prepositioned epistemic hedge. *Research on Language & Social Interaction, 44*(4), 317–337.

Whalen, M. R., & Zimmerman, D. H. (1987). Sequential and institutional contexts in calls for help. *Social Psychology Quarterly, 50*(2), 172–185.

Whalen, M. R., & Zimmerman, D. H. (1990). Describing trouble: Practical epistemology in citizen calls to the police. *Language in Society, 19*(4), 465–492.

Whalen, J., Zimmerman, D. H., & Whalen, M. (1988). When words fail: A single case analysis. *Social Problems, 35*(4), 335–362.

Zimmerman, D. H. (1984). Talk and its occasions: The case of calling the police. In D. Schiffrin (Ed.), *Meaning, form, and use in context: Linguistic applications. Georgetown University roundtable on language and linguistics* (pp. 210–228). Georgetown University Press.

Zimmerman, D. H. (1992a). Achieving context: Openings in emergency calls. In G. Watson & R. M. Seiler (Eds.), *Text in context: Contributions to ethnomethodology* (pp. 35–51). Sage.

Zimmerman, D. H. (1992b). The interactional organization of calls for emergency assistance. In P. Drew & J. Heritage (Eds.), *Talk at work: Social interaction in institutional settings* (pp. 418–469). Cambridge University Press.

CHAPTER 6

When There Is a Language Issue

Abstract This chapter deals with language difficulties in emergency calls due to the fact that the caller is not a speaker of the call-taker's language and that the call-taker does not understand the caller's language. Using a single case analysis, I focus on a call where a professional interpreter is sought. I describe the language trouble between caller and call-taker, the ways in which the professional interpreter was recruited, the conversation of the interpreter with the caller and the interpreter's rendering of the caller's need. I argue that the work of the interpreter is less than that of a translation machine and more than that of the coordinator of meanings and understandings.

Keywords Language barriers • Interpreting work • Professional translation service • Interpreter's renditions • Narratives

1 Emergency Calls and Language Barriers

One of the many challenges facing healthcare today consists of the cultural and linguistic barriers in health communication that affect healthcare access and quality. Studies on the employment of intercultural mediators and interpreters in healthcare demonstrate that difficulties associated with speakers with limited language proficiency are best overcome with the use of a professional interpreter who can ensure good communication between

G. Fele, *Emergency Communication*,
https://doi.org/10.1007/978-3-031-26239-5_6

patients and healthcare professionals (Haffner, 1992). But there are no easy solutions to language barrier problems in the access to health services, and we still need better knowledge on how communication matters in the encounters between professionals and patients with limited language proficiency. As Jacobs et al. (2006) have noted, there is a "need for more research on language barriers in health care".

If communication is of great importance for patient safety and quality care in examinations by general practitioners or in hospitals, it is all more so for emergency services, and in particular during the handling of emergency calls (Gerwing & Indseth, 2016). Difficulties associated with limited language proficiency can seriously hamper efforts to collect accurate and timely information on what has happened and where. In order to send the help most appropriate for the case at hand, emergency operators typically rely on the adequacy, precision and reliability of the initial report of the emergency event. Such descriptions are the product of joint interactional work between the caller and the emergency operator (Heritage & Clayman, 2010; Cromdal, 2012). Moreover, time is a critical factor in the handling of emergency calls. Emergency services come increasingly under strain because of language barriers, for a series of reasons: the growing numbers of tourists and visitors from foreign countries; the growing presence of immigrants; the complex composition of the population, as in South Africa where 11 official languages are currently spoken, together with other indigenous or local languages (Penn et al., 2017). Emergency call conversations are sometimes conducted with limited and unequally distributed language skills (Osvaldsson et al., 2013). Persons in distress may find it difficult to make their needs clear and consequently seek assistance from another party to make the call. In some families or homes for the elderly, where the care is often left to caregivers or personal assistants from other countries, the caller may be someone who lacks the appropriate language skills or is not comfortable in making the call. In order to overcome these difficulties in communication management, interpreters' services have been installed at emergency call centres in several countries.

An increasing number of studies have examined emergency calls in the case of a language barrier. One line of inquiry assesses the effect of language barriers on dispatching (time and efficacy) compared with calls where the caller speaks the same language as the call-taker (Meischke et al.,

2013).[1] Even if this line of research is plausible, it necessarily concentrates only on the outcomes of the call and risks, overlooking the way in which language barriers matter *during actual calls*. Moreover, the meaning itself of language barrier is too often taken for granted. Meischke et al. (2013, p. 476) observed, "Telecommunicators are trained to note a language barrier whenever they experience difficulty communicating with a caller due to the caller's lack of English fluency." But what exactly call-takers consider to be a language barrier has gone unexplored and what kind of communication challenges arise in the management of an emergency call has not been analysed. From my point of view, a useful starting point is to consider the ways in which some communicative problems end up being considered a 'language barrier' *by the participants*. It has been documented that for a large majority of emergency calls where there is a language mismatch, it is handled smoothly and does not cause any disruption (Penn et al., 2017). Second, what is under-analysed is that a communicative problem due to a lack of language proficiency is often remedied by the participants in many different ways. A communicative problem due to the fact that people engaged in some kind of mutual interaction have no language in common can be handled by the participants with different semiotic resources—or if only spoken language is used, with some kind of "linguistic minestrone" (Burke, 2006, p. 108)—in order to maximize understanding and minimize the chance of there not being even the slightest comprehension (but, obviously, thus increasing the likelihood of misunderstanding[2]). This may be the very pragmatic response by people when some kind of linguistic difficulty is encountered. They try to mobilize all their linguistic resources (drawn from even different languages) in order to overcome a real obstacle to communication. Osvaldsson et al. (2013), on analysing an emergency call from a 12-year-old who was not hearably a native speaker of the language of the national emergency service (Swedish), well evidenced two features of non-native/native communication in such a case: first, the attention paid to possible problems of comprehension, in order to anticipate any obstacles to mutual understanding; second, the systematic deployment by the call-taker of repair methods (repeating elements of the

[1] For instance, in terms of on-scene upgrades and on-scene downgrades of the severity of emergency codes attributed to calls with language barriers compared with ordinary calls (Meischke et al., 2013).

[2] See Gerwing and Indseth (2016) for a plea to instruct operators to improve and develop their own communication skills with non-native callers.

previous turn difficult to understand for the call-taker; presenting alternative ways to give information; or postponing problematic exchanges to later stages of the call). In cases like this one, participants use all their interactional resources in order to proceed with the call and to ensure that mutual comprehension has been achieved. Svennevig et al. (2019) conducted a quantitative analysis of simulated emergency calls and analysed pre-emptive strategies (such as reformulations, simplifications, etc.) used by first-language speakers in talk addressed to second-language speakers in order to minimize problems of understanding.

Only when difficult communication is systematically and definitively hampering the 'progressivity' (Stivers & Robinson, 2006) of the interactional encounter is a 'language barrier' in place. Hence, a linguistic problem is often more a matter of degree than a radical interruption of the communicative flow in the social fabric of interaction.

In regard to the ways in which the linguistic problem is dealt with in emergency calls, it has been observed how callers and dispatchers relate to each other so as to maximize understanding. In the case of linguistic problems due to the fact that the caller speaks a language different from that of the call-taker, there are solid grounds for arguing that all the communicative resources at hand are exploited in order to keep the communication going. These contextual or ad hoc communicative resources appear to be arranged in a sequence of options. Firstly, the call-takers endeavour to see whether the two (call-taker *and* caller) can understand each other with their own communicative (linguistic) resources. Secondly, if the first option fails to yield the expected results, the call-taker and the caller can look for an occasional interpreter, someone who—in the call centre or close to the caller—can act as an interpreter. Only if also this second option fails will the call-taker ask for a professional interpreter, which is thus the third and last option. Appeal to an interpreting service is only the last resort (Emerson, 1981): and this happens only when the callers present themselves "in a way which evidences that they are incapable of conducting the call" in the language of the call-taker (Raymond, 2014a). This observation matches the finding of Meischke et al. (2010): even if for the call-takers interviewed in their research, the primary strategy for communication with LEP (Limited English Proficiency) callers was the use of a telephone interpreter line known as the Language Line, it was utilized in only 13% of LEP calls.

Raymond (2014a) pointed out that, before the caller is switched to an external interpreting service, the call-taker and the caller negotiate the use of the language in the very first sequence of the call.[3] On the basis of a corpus of 97 calls from Spanish speakers to a 911 call centre in the United States, Raymond showed that there were no calls where there was an immediate transfer to a translation service: "on the contrary, call-takers consistently respond to all forms of language requests with a bid for English" (Raymond, 2014a, p. 41). There are good reasons for this reluctance on the part of call-takers to use professional interpretation services in managing emergency calls. As also emerges from the literature, there are some counter-indications for using a professional interpreter in an emergency call. Most of the *time delay* associated with language barrier calls can be attributed to the use of interpretation services (Meischke et al., 2013). When an interpretation service is used, the call-taker must trade off the potential for clarity and accuracy in the communication with the additional time taken to access and allow for interpretation (Meischke et al., 2013). In general, although call-takers may access over-the-phone interpreter (OPI) services to facilitate communication, managing three-way communication during an emergency is challenging. As Carroll et al. (2013) pointed out, there is little published research on the relationship between LEP callers and call-takers and on the role of OPI services during these calls. Meischke et al. (2010) cursorily observed that LEP callers received more repetition, rephrasing and slowing of speech than the non-LEP callers, but they did not provide any systematic analysis of how such calls are managed. Furthermore, little is known about effective strategies to manage such calls. I concur with the conclusion drawn by Meischke et al. (2010) that more research should be conducted on 'best practices' for phone-based emergency communication with LEP callers. What is required in particular is an analysis of actual phone calls, given that at present most research is based on questionnaires (Carroll et al., 2013; Meischke et al., 2013; Kale et al., Kale & Syed, 2010; Meischke et al., 2010) or secondary analysis of cohort data (Bradley et al., 2011), or on qualitative data which lack the details of actual talk (Meischke et al., 2013; Ong et al., 2012). In any case, relying on an interpreting service is not an easy solution to the language barrier. Still to be studied are the processes and mechanisms of communication whereby emergency calls are handled through an interpreting service. This chapter is a step forward in this direction.

[3] See Rasmussen et al. (2002) study on international phone calls, where they note that "the potential fragility of an international telephone conversation is established in the first turn of the caller" (p. 128).

2 What Is a Language Barrier and How Is It Dealt with by the Participants?

I examine a single case (Schegloff, 1987; Whalen et al., 1988) of a call to an emergency call centre that ended with recourse to an interpreting service. I shall first analyse in what ways a language barrier is recognized as such by the speakers—call-taker and caller alike. Second, I will consider the contact of the call-taker with the interpreting service. Third, I will analyse interpreting as a mediation work between the caller and the call-taker.

I begin with the incoming call to the PSAP:

Excerpt 6.1 Wir Sind Hier Im Hotel

```
02 Ctaker    centodiciotto:
             one one eight:
03 Caller    ja, Sie sprechen deutsch?
             yes, do you speak German?
04 Ctaker    tz, no.
             tz, no
05 Caller    ä::h,
             ä::h,
06           wir sind hier im, im hotel
             we are here at, at the hotel
07           wai-
             wai-
08 ???       NOME ALBERGO ((in the background))
             HOTEL NAME
09 Caller    NOME ALBERGO
             HOTEL NAME
10 Ctaker    tz, no no, e::h, italiano,
             tz, no no, e::h, Italian,
11           c'è qualcuno che parla italiano
             is there anyone who speaks Italian
```

In this excerpt, the caller produces a request for language in line 3, in her very first turn. As we have repeatedly seen, the turn immediately following identification of the service by the call-taker is occupied by the caller as she/he states the problem for which she/he has contacted the emergency number. In this case, by contrast, some kind of language issue is immediately put forward by the caller before the presentation of the problem and the request for assistance (line 3: *ja, Sie sprechen deutsch?—yes, do you speak German?*). This is a direct request (Raymond, 2014a) to use a language that is not the one of the call-taker. The call-taker responds negatively with a direct or type-conforming answer (Raymond, 2003), without any bids for Italian. This is the first moment in which the absence of a common language is apparent. It is the very first place where a linguistic asymmetry between caller and call-taker emerges. This linguistic diversity immediately becomes a problem: the call-taker does not speak the language of the caller. It is at this point that a first communication barrier arises.

But this is not the end of the call. The participants negotiate how to continue. For both the call-taker and the caller, the problem is how to proceed. A first solution is provided by the caller. After initial uncertainty, the caller simply continues talking. In her language (German), the caller begins to describe the problem for which she wants assistance, starting to give a first description of the place "they" are *(wir sind hier im, im hotel,—we are here at, at the hotel ...*, lines 6–8). Continuing to talk and see what happens is a first strategy to overcome the communication block: the call-taker may perhaps understand some German, or he may have someone nearby who speaks German, or he could find yet another solution not available to the caller.

Just after this point, the communication problem is exposed and made evident. The call-taker cannot follow the caller in her language and asks to talk in his language, Italian (line 10: *tz, no no, e::h, Italiano—no no, Italian*). It is possible to overhear on the line (line 8 of the transcript) someone close to the caller whom she addresses and who is suggesting the name of the hotel. This is a sign for the call-taker that there may be someone nearby who speaks Italian (and German) and could be of help in being the interpreter (line 11: *c'è qualcuno che parla italiano?—is there anyone who speaks Italian*).

In sum, we have observed the turn-by-turn push for Italian "in search of sufficient grounds on which to turn down callers' request for" non-Italian (Raymond, 2014a, p. 53). The call-taker is aware that the caller has no knowledge of Italian but at the same time seeks any means to see if the call can be continued in Italian—in this case noticing that there is someone nearby who can be used as a language bridge.

The following excerpt shows that it is possible to observe a sequence beginning with similar language problem but with a different solution to the language problem:

Excerpt 6.2 How Good Is Your English (A)

01	Ctaker	centodiciotto pronto
		one one eight hello
02	Caller	hallo? (can you- eh)
03		is there someone who speaks English, please?
04	Ctaker	eh number *ambulance*.
05		krankenwagen ((ambulance in German))
06	Caller	ya, well,
07		I we- I have gone up the mountain with my friend
08		and, he has been struck by lightning.
09	Ctaker	eh serve *ambulance*? ((ambulance in English))
		do you need ambulance
10	Caller	eh (we- we are) we are on the track to ( )
11		he is able to walk but ( )
12	Ctaker	sei bona a parlare inglese? ((to a colleague nearby))
		how good is your English?
13		((the colleague nods and takes her earphones))
14		ein moment. ((in German))
		one moment.
15	Caller	okay, thank you

The caller's first turn is initially designed to express a direct request for help (line 3: *can you-*), which is suddenly stopped, to be turned into a direct request for a language—this time for English (line 3: *is there someone who speaks English, please?*). In this case, the call-taker does not answer in the negative but provides a sort of confirmation that the caller has reached the right number, that of the emergency call centre, albeit in a sort of 'language minestrone' mixing broken English and German (lines 4–5: *number ambulance, kranken wagen*). This is taken by the caller as an invitation to go ahead, provided that the call-taker's turn embodies some knowledge of English. The caller states the reason for the call: that is, a description of what has happened (lines 7–8: *I we- I have gone up the mountain with my friend and, he has been struck by lightning*). The call-taker's reply makes explicit what the description of the fact implies—a request for help (line 9: *serve ambulance [in English]—do you need an ambulance?*)—again using some English, suggesting that the call can be continued using the language of the caller. After the caller continues to provide details about the place and the condition of his friend (lines 10–11: *we are on the track to ((incomprehensible)), he can walk but ( ))*, the call-taker turns to his colleague in the room (line 12: *sei bona a parlare inglese?—how good is your English?*). Having secured the collaboration of his colleague, the call-taker turns to the caller using a German expression (that can be easily recognized also by an English speaker), *ein moment* (line 14), putting a hold on the call. The caller acknowledges the call-taker's turn and expresses gratitude for taking care of the language problem (line 15 : *okay, thank you*).

Let us see what happens with this new round of exchange in this call with a different call-taker.

Excerpt 6.3 How Good Is Your English (B)—Continuation of Excerpt 6.2

16		(4.0)
17	Ctaker	hallo?
18	Caller	hallo?
19	Ctaker	yes
20	Caller	(do-) do you understand English?
21	Ctaker	a little bit
22	Caller	yes
23	Ctaker	okay
24	Caller	we are-, we- we are on the mountain,
25		we are on ah (Mount) Altissimo

The call-taker's opening turn (line 17: *hallo*) that resumes the call is in English, as is the call-taker's confirmation that the call has restarted (line 19: *yes*). Before resuming the call from where it has been suspended, the caller inquires about the call-taker's capacity regarding the language that is used to ask for help (line 20: *do you understand English?*). Note that the first language knowledge check was made in terms of 'speaking' the language, whereas this second check is made in terms of 'understanding' it. Apparent here is a de-escalating expectation regarding the call-taker's proficiency level. In any case, the call-taker's confirmation (line 21: *a little bit*) is a clear sign for the caller to go ahead in the call with a description of the place where the accident has happened (lines 2425: *we are on the mountain, we are on Mount Altissimo*[4]).

[4] Monte Altissimo at Nago (2079 m) forms part of the Garda pre-Alps and specifically the Monte Baldo range. There is a beautiful view of Lake Garda from its summit.

In sum, we have seen how the caller took samples of language different from Italian as a sign to continue using English during the call, assuming that the call-taker had enough language competence to understand English. The call-taker then handed the call over to a nearby colleague, and the call could continue in English on the assumption that the call-taker 'understood' rather than 'spoke' English.

3 Turning to a Professional Translation Service

In the rest of the chapter, I consider more ordinary interactional problems that arise when the assistance of a professional interpreter is sought.

Let us go back to what happened in the first call that we examined. The call-taker was able to talk to the person near the German caller, but she revealed that she knew nothing about what had happened, and that she was unable to ask the caller anything because she actually did not speak any German. It was at this point that the call-taker decided to call the professional translation service. Below is an excerpt from the contact call with the professional translation service:

Excerpt 6.4 Turning to a Professional Interpreter

```
01 Ctaker   pronto:?
            hello?
02 Interp   pronto?
            hello?
03 Ctaker   sì è il cento[diciotto
            yes this is one one eight
04 Interp                [sì pronto
                          yes hello
05          buongiorno
            good morning
06 Ctaker   è il centodiciotto, buongiorno
            this is one one eight, good morning
07          (2.8)
08          pronto:::
            hello:::
09 Interp   sì pronto buongiorno
            yes hello good morning
10 Ctaker   mi sente:?
            can you hear me?
```

(*continued*)

Excerpt 6.4 (continued)

```
11          (2.0)
12 Interp   sì, benissimo, sì
            yes, very clear, yes
13 Ctaker   occhei. è il centodiciotto, la centrale operativa
            okay. this is one one eight, operation centre
14          (1.4)
15          REGIONE  emergen[za
            REGIONAL emergency
16 Interp                   [sì
                             yes
17          (2.2)
18          sì
            yes
19 Ctaker   ecco avrei bisogno di una traduzione::
            okay I would need a translation
20          mhm tedesco.
            mhm German.
21          per delle persone che chiamano [da [CITTA]
            for  people  calling     from CITY NAME
22 Interp                                      [sì sì
                                                 yes yes
23 Ctaker   e mi serve sapere dov-, eh,
            and I need to know where: eh
24          sapere dove si trova la persona e cosa è successo
            to know where the person is and what has happened
25          (1.4)
26 Interp   occhei
            okay
27 Ctaker   d'accordo?
            okay?
28          (2.2)
29 Interp   sì
            yes
30 Ctaker   rimanga in linea eh?
            hold on eh?
            (1.6)
31 Interp   occhei
            okay
```

This is the call between the call-taker and the professional translation service where the call-taker gives instructions to the interpreter. To be noted is the general organization of this kind of call into three parts: the first part is devoted to reciprocal identification (a rather long sequence: lines 1–18); the second part is occupied by the instructions that the call-taker gives to the interpreter (lines 19–29); the third part concerns the switching of the translation service to the caller (lines 30–31).

We focus on the second part of the sequence. The call-taker frames the request in terms of the need for translation, specifying the language requested (German) (lines 19–20). The call-taker asks the interpreter to inquire where the caller is calling from and the reason for the call (line 24: *to know where the person is and what has happened*). The caller is asking the interpreter to act as the call-taker would act if there was not a language issue. What is interesting is that the call-taker does not give the interpreter any information regarding what to do after she has collected the information requested. The interpreter is left with the task of asking questions, but she has no idea if the answer is appropriate and when the answer should be considered completed.

I concur with the view of Baraldi and Gavioli (2012, see also Gavioli and Baraldi, 2011) that interpreting work consists of coordinating the production of meaning in social interaction. What is interesting is that many studies on the uses of translation services in healthcare focus only on the actual work of 'rendering' (the translation from one language to another), and deal with issues concerning the reliability, faithfulness and trustworthiness of the translation. However, this approach overlooks the fact that a large part of an interpreter's work involves 'non-renditions': that is, coordinating participation in the conversation and its organization. In this regard, what should be considered is how a complex interaction among three parties, two of them not sharing the same linguistic resources, develops under a strong temporal constraint.

4 The Interpreter's Work

Let us consider the work of the interpreter. We have shown the first moments of the phone call in which the interpreter was instructed on her task. In particular, the call-taker told the interpreter to ask the caller about 'what had happened' and 'where it had happened', which are the items of information essential for handling an emergency.

Excerpt 6.5 Helpvoice Interpreting School Contacting the Caller

44	Interp	hallo
		hello
45	Caller	ja
		yes
46	Interp	guten morgen
		good morning
47		ich bin NAME von der Dolmetscherschule von HelpVoice
		this is NAME from the HelpVoice interpreting school
48	Caller	ah
		ah
49	Interp	Sie sollen mir bitte sagen was passiert ist
		please tell me what has happened
50		und wo Sie sich befinden
		and where you are
51	Caller	ja, wir sind hier in diesem Hotel ( )
		well, we are here in this hotel ( )

The interpreter is finally connected to the caller. After introducing herself (lines 44–48), she translates almost literally into German[5] the requests previously made by the call-taker in Italian (*could you please tell me what has happened and where you are*, lines 49–50). The two questions are worded to elicit an expanded answer in response, especially in regard to definition of the problem for which the caller has contacted the emergency service. The interpreter's questions are not formatted in the third person (e.g., "could you tell the call-taker…") and the caller is supposed to address the interpreter directly as the recipient of the answer.

4.1 *The Caller's Narrative*

After the initial questions by the interpreter, the caller starts to reply. The answer is a rather elaborate one, and it develops over several turns, generating a long sequence.

[5] Moreover, in the interpreter's turn there is a politeness marker "bitte" ("please") (line 49) that would be strange to find in requests formulated by call-takers.

Excerpt 6.6 Caller's Narrative in German to the Interpreter

```
51 Caller   ja, wir sind hier in diesem hotel (     )
            well, we are here in this hotel (     )
52 ??       NOME HOTEL
            HOTEL NAME
53 Caller   NOME HOTEL
            HOTEL NAME
54          a::h und-, a:h=
            a::h e-, a:h=
55 Interp   =ja=
            =yes=
56 Caller   =wir sind mitn bus da
            we came by bus
57          (1.0)
58          wir sind mit einem reisebus da im im hotel NAME
            we arrived by bus at at the hotel NAME
59          in ä::h ca- cabri (     )
            in e::h ca- cabri (     )
60 Interp   ja
            yes
61 Caller   und wir haben jetzt ne frau,
            there is a woman
62          di::e ist heute aufgewacht und weiß nimmer,
            who woke up today and doesn´t remember
63          wie sie her gekommen ist,
            how she arrived here,
64          ä:h und
            e:h e
65 Interp   oke
            okay
66 Caller   ja, ich- ich habe einen verdacht auf in m
            yes, I- I suspect she has had m
67 Interp   ja
            yes
68 Caller   in-, ja infarkt
            heart attack
```

(*continued*)

Excerpt 6.6 (continued)

```
69              °hhh ä:h sch[laganfall
                °hhh a:h stroke
70 Interp                   [(.....)
71 Caller       so was in die richtung, eh?
                something like this, eh?
72 Interp       mhm m
73 Caller       und ich mein [sie ist zwar ansprechbar alles
                and I think, even if she is reactive to everything
74 Interp                    [oke
                              okay
75 Calle        ä:h aber sie wusste gar net
                e:h but she doesn´t remember
76              ob sie ihre tabletten genommen ha, sie weiß-
                if she has taken her pills, she doesn't-
77 Interp       oke
                okay
78 Caller       und sie weiß nicht, wie sie her gekommen ist
                and she doesn´t know how she has arrived
79 Interp       mhm
80 Caller       und es ist mir einfach zu ge[fährlich
                honestly it seems to be too dangerous
81 Interp                                   [oke
                                             okay
82 Caller       ich bin kinderkran[kenschwester
                I am a child nurse
83 Interp                         [ja
                                   yes
84 Caller       und kenn mich insofern da aus
                and for this I am familiar with these things
85              NOME HOTEL?
                HOTEL NAME?
86 Caller       ja
                yes
87 Interp       wo wo ist das genau das hotel?
                where is the hotel exactly?
88 Caller       es ist ganz oben am berg in in Wika- ka
                it´s just up the mountain at at Vika -ka
```

(*continued*)

Excerpt 6.6 (continued)

```
89 Interp   ah.
90          haben Sie die adresse, vielleicht die genaue
            do you have the exact address
91          die Sie mir sagen können.
            that you can give me.
92 Caller   des ä::h muss Ihnen die die die das mädel selber sagen
            the girl could tell it to you
93          weil ich weiß nicht wie wir her gekommen sind
            because I don´t know how we reached here
94 Interp   oke
            okay
95 Caller   wir sind wir sind gestern
            we came here yesterday
96          in der tiefsten finsternis hier angekommen
            in the deepest darkness
97          ((laugh))
98          ich weiß bloß, dass wir-
            I only know that we-
99 Interp   oke, (alles)
            okay, (all)
100 Caller  sagen Sie, wo wir woh[nen, das hotel? ((to ??))
            can you say where we are, the hotel
101 Interp                       [alles klar
                                  all clear
102 Caller  sagen Sie bitte wo das hotel ist, bitte ((a C2))
            can you say please where the hotel is ((to C2))
103 Interp  (pronto) allora, la:: ((to the call-taker))
            (hello) well, the
104         la signora è la la guida turistica di un
            the lady is the the tourist guide of a
105         di un bus turistico
            of a tourist bus
106 Ctaker  sì
            yes
```

As can be seen, it takes more than 50 lines to transcribe the answers to two questions. Let us review what happens in this long sequence.

The caller begins her turn by giving the name of the hotel (lines 51–53), with the help of a person near to her (line 52). The caller first gives a short definition of the place where "they" are located (lines 51–53, where the "we are" used by the caller instead of "I am" projects that the caller is not asking for help for herself but for someone else), and then begins to describe the problem. Just after stating the location, the caller produces a hesitation (line 54) which can be interpreted as a prompt for instructions on what to do next (should I go on or wait?). The interpreter's subsequent turn tells the caller what kind of sequence will ensue.

The interpreter produces an item (line 55: *ja*, *yes*) that confirms what has been said just before by the caller and invites the caller to continue producing her turn. The caller has hesitated (line 54) after providing the first information requested (regarding where they are), and she indicates uncertainty to the interpreter as to how the conversation can proceed. The interpreter's turn ("yes") signals to the caller that she can proceed. The interpreter thus tacitly instructs the caller that the interpreter is not going to give a translation step by step. The caller is instructed to continue; no further questions or requests for clarification are provided by the interpreter at this point. No immediate referral of information by the interpreter to the call-taker is made. The interpreter invites the caller to add new pieces of information. The caller is instructed on the fact that she will not be interrupted in her narrative.

The caller's definition of the problem starts with a narrative. She begins to provide details on the event, starting with those that appear to be the antecedents of the problem itself (line 56: *we came by bus*, which is fully expanded in lines 58–59 after a pause that has not been used by the interpreter to stop the narrative or to simply take the floor back). The interpreter produces an acknowledgement token (line 60: *yes*), again inviting the caller to proceed with her description. Just after this second acknowledgement by the interpreter, the caller produces what can be considered the first full formulation of the problem (lines 61–63: *there is a woman who woke up today and doesn't remember how she arrived here*).

This is the first point in the conversation where the interpreter could have turned to the call-taker with a rendition of the problem because here it appears that the two questions have received a possible complete answer. What instead happens is that the interpreter produces another acknowledgement token (line 64: *okay* with rising intonation, immediately after the caller has produced the first formulation of the problem and expresses uncertainty cues regarding what to do next). With the acknowledgement token, the interpreter invites the caller to go ahead and provide further items in description of the problem. From this point onwards, an extensive narrative of facts gradually develops (lines 66–80). It is made possible and elicited by the interpreter, who at several junctures of the conversation produces further continuers (lines 67, 70, 72, 74, 77, 79, 81, 83).

The caller's narrative is interrupted by the interpreter with a question again regarding the hotel, asking for its exact name and address (lines 90–91). This is information that the caller does not know; the third person nearby is asked to produce it for the interpreter (lines 92–93, and 100). With the *alles klar* (*all clear*) at line 101, the interpreter signals that she has collected all the information requested. This turn marks the end of the caller's narrative. It is at this point that the interpreter addresses the call-taker for the first time (lines 103–105), and she offers to render into Italian what has been collected thus far.

What we have seen are some features of the interpreter's work in an emergency call. The question that we have addressed is this: At what point should the caller's turn be considered completed—that is, should be considered by the interpreter as a relevant and exhaustive answer to the question asked by the call-taker? The ways in which the interpreter enables the production of a patient's long turns is the topic of a very interesting article by Gavioli (2012). But Gavioli does not address the issue of the relevance of the patient's long turns for medical purposes: that is, when a narrative should be considered as complete or adequate as a possible answer to a doctor's question. Here the question is this: At what point of the caller's narrative can the interpreter turn to the call-taker and give a rendition of the information collected thus far? Can the interpreter enter into the caller's narrative to obtain further details that may specify an otherwise vague description? Who decides what a vague description is: the interpreter or the call-taker? Who decides what details may be relevant to management of the emergency? Can the simple fact that the caller may stop her description (i.e., not add further details) be considered an appropriate slot for the interpreter to turn to the call-taker to render what has been collected thus far? Or can the interpreter invite the caller to continue to furnish additional items of information? Who controls the conversation: the interpreter or the call-taker? What are the responsibilities of the interpreter? The interpreter is in a position, at any juncture of the conversation, to evaluate the completeness, consistency and satisfactoriness of the information received. In short, the interpreter must make decisions at every point of the call that affect important aspects of the call-taker's professional work.

4.2 *The Interpreter's Rendition*

Now we consider the rendition work by the interpreter. As we have seen, the overall situation is rather complicated: the call-taker has asked a professional translation service to talk in German to a woman who has called the emergency call centre not for herself but for another woman. Close to the calling woman, there is another woman (presumably a member of the hotel staff), who speaks Italian and who does not speak German, but who is assisting the caller with small items of simple, even if vital, information (such as the full name of the hotel). Once the basic information requested by the call-taker has been collected (Excerpt 6.4, line 24: *where the person is and what has happened*), the interpreter turns back to the call-taker to refer.

As the collection of the information from the caller turned out to be a narrative, so the rendition of the information by the interpreter to the call-taker turned into a narrative as well.

Excerpt 6.7 Interpreter Rendition to the Call-taker

```
103 Interp  (pronto) allora, la::
            (hello) well, the
104         la signora è la la guida turistica di un
            the lady is the the tourist guide of a
105         di un bus turistico
            of a tourist bus
106 Ctaker  sì
            yes
107 Interp  e::h sono arrivati ieri eh e stamattina una signora
            e::h they arrived yesterday eh e this morning a lady
108         che fa parte del gruppo si è [svegliata e:
            who is part of the group got up and
109 Ctaker                               [sì
                                          yes
110 Interp  on non, non sapeva come è arrivata
            she didn't know how she had arrived
111         e non sapeva ni[ente
            and she didn't know anything
112 Ctaker                 [m
```

(*continued*)

Excerpt 6.7 (continued)

```
113 Interp   qu[indi
             so
114 Ctaker     [hm
115 Interp   hanno, hanno il sospetto di un di un ictus.
             they suspect she has had a stroke.
116 Ctaker   ho capito.
             I've understood.
117          ma adesso parla male::,
             but does she speak poorly now,
118          muove: le braccia le gambe
             does she move her arms her legs
119          le muove tutte:: le (...)
             does she move all of them: (...)
120 Interp   no no, se:, no no, e:h, e:h assolutamente m,
             no no, if:, no no, e:h, e:h absolutely m,
121          sì può parlare ma eh
             yes she can speak but eh
122          non ricorda nulla.
             she doesn't remember anything.
123 Ctaker   (    )
124 Interp   non sa: se ha preso le: le: le medicinali, quindi
             she doesn't know if she has taken her medicine, so
125 Ctaker   [occhei,
              okay
126 Interp   [m
127 Ctaker   e nah-, e ha capito
             and, did you understand
             se è una persona [anziana?
             if she is an elderly person?
128 Interp                    [e l'albergo
                               and the hotel's
129          si chiama albergo albergo NOME
             name is hotel hotel NAME
130 Ctaker   NOME ALBERGO sì quello l'aveva detto prima
             HOTEL'S NAME yes she has already told me,
```

(*continued*)

Excerpt 6.7 (continued)

131		la: la:, la signora.
		the lady.
132		e::::h, è una perso[na anziana?
		e::::h, is she an elderly person?
133	Interp	[ah
134	Ctaker	ve l'ha detto?
		did she tell you
135		(3.0)
136	Interp	hören Sie mich noch? ((to the caller))
		do you still hear me?

The interpreter's onset turn to the call-taker gains his attention by being in Italian (line 103: *(pronto), allora, (hello), so*). This turn in Italian furnishes an initial description of who the caller is (lines 104–105: *the lady is a tourist guide of a tourist bus*). The call-taker replies with a confirmation token (line 106: *yes*) just after this first item of information, and the interpreter goes ahead with the story, from which emerges the problem in need of help.

The description of the problem is an almost word-by-word rendition of what the interpreter has gathered in the conversation with the caller: the description of facts (*a lady who is part of the group, got up*, and *she didn't know how she had arrived*, lines 107–108 and 110), and their interpretation (*they suspect she has had a stroke*, line 115). The story is an example of indirect reported speech, *where the speaker summarizes or conveys the words of another without purporting to enact them* (Holt, 2017, p. 171). The call-taker is advised that the call for help is being made on behalf of a third party, and he sustains the interpreter's rendition with sequentially positioned understanding tokens that invite the interpreter to continue the story (lines 109 *yes*, 112 *m*, 114 *hm*). The production of an explicit understanding turn (line 116 *I've understood*) marks the end of the rendition.

The call-taker then asks the interpreter for additional information regarding the state of the patient (lines 117–118 *does she speak poorly, does she move her arms legs*), elements of the situation that were not included in the first rendition (Raymond, 2014b). The questions are addressed to the interpreter and consider the interpreter as a knowledgeable person, entitled to answer (there is no sign of modifiers such as "do you know if", or "did you ask if"). The interpreter herself provides the answer (lines 120–124: *no no, absolutely, yes, she can speak but she doesn't remember anything, she doesn't know if she has taken her medicine*). The interpreter does not turn to the caller to have the answer from her, showing that the information requested was already collected in the previous conversation with the caller.

The call-taker closes with an *okay* (line 125) (Mondada & Sorjonen, 2021) the previous question-answer sequence with the interpreter, marking at the same time that he has understood the prior information and that it was not enough to have a complete picture (some new information or action was registered but indexed as not yet complete for local practical concerns, Betz & Deppermann, 2021, p. 83). The call-taker, in fact, asks another question, this time addressing the interpreter not as a depository of the information but as the person who has collected information from another source (line 127: ***did you understand*** *if she is an elderly person?*—emphasis mine). After an exchange about the name of the hotel where the emergency is located, the call-taker repeats the question (lines 132–134: *is she an elderly person? did she tell you?*), making apparent in his turn that this is a piece of information that is needed.

After a pause (line 135) the interpreter addresses the caller directly in German, with no signs that she is moving from one conversant to another. She is going to inquire the caller regarding the information requested by the call-taker.

4.3 Interpreter's Initiatives

So far, we have analysed the interpreter's work in an emergency call not from a purely linguistic point of view (i.e., how she/he can provide a reliable rendering), but from the social interaction perspective. In particular, it is interesting to consider the multiple ways in which an interpreter can be more than just a "sounding box" (Goffman, 1979, p. 16) and can take initiatives that depart from what can be naively expected to be the work of interpreting.

Let us turn to the last excerpt examined in this chapter, that of the second round of conversation between the interpreter and the caller.

Excerpt 6.8 Interpreter Talking for the Second Time with the Caller

```
132 Ctaker  e::::h, è una perso[na anziana?
            e::::h, is she an elderly person?
133 Interp                     [ah
134 Ctaker  ve l'ha detto?
            did she tell you
135         (3.0)
136 Interp  hören Sie mich noch?
            do you still hear me?
      ...
     ((3 lines omitted))
      ...
140 Caller  hallo
            hello
141         (2.0)
142 Interp  ja, a:h ist die, wie alt ist die frau ungefähr?
            yes, so approximately, how old is the woman?
143 Caller  och Gott, sechzig also wenn (     )
            good Lord, around sixty?
144 Interp  ja aber net so hochbetagt nicht?
            so, not really old?
145 Caller  nein normal ist die noch fit, und und ja
            no, normally she is in really good health
146 Interp  oke und, und hat sie irgendwie das gesicht verzogen
            okay, and is there something distorted in her face
147         oder bewegt sie sich schlecht oder, oder?
            or does she move badly, or something like that?
148 Caller  nein sie sie ist ansprechbar, aber sie ist eben von
            no, she is responsive, but she is just
149         ihren gedanken her. ne? weiß sie nimmer
            with her thoughts. right?, she doesn't ((remember))
150 Interp  =allora
            =well
151 Ctaker  sì, sì, dimmi.
            yes, yes, tell me.
```

(continued)

Excerpt 6.8 (continued)

```
152 Interp la signora ha sì uhm sessantasett'anni ma è-
           the lady is sixty-seven years old but she is-
       ...
       ((3 lines omitted))
       ...
156 Interp e::h, s:-, diciamo sessantacinque anni e::
           e::h, s:-, let's say sixty-five and::
157 Ctaker [occhei
           okay
158 Interp [è abbastanza (   ) sana come un, come un pesce.
           she's fit as a, as a fiddle.
159 Ctaker sì
           yes
```

The excerpt begins where the previous one ended, with the call-taker asking the interpreter if the caller has given information about the patient's age (lines 132–134: *is she an elderly person? Did she tell you?*). The interpreter resumes talking in German to the caller (line 136: *do you still hear me?*), and then asks about the patient's age (line 142: *so how old is the woman?*). Observe that the call-taker's question asked if the patient was an elderly person, whereas the interpreter's question is how old she is: the two questions projected two different answers. After receiving the answer to her question (line 143: *well, Jesus, around sixty?*), the interpreter advances a guess in terms of the type of question asked by the call-taker (*so, not really old*, line 144). This guess is taken by the caller to be a comment on the age of the patient (not a way to translate and conform the caller's answer to the type of question put by the call-taker), and as under reserve about the description of the situation that could cast doubt on the seriousness of the request for help. The interpreter's turn engenders a reply by the caller (*no, usually she's in really good health*, line 145), which implies that, even if the patient is not an elderly person, the fact that she is usually in good health and now seems confused makes the call for help reasonable.

The interpreter then asks the caller another question (*is there something distorted or does she move her face badly, or something like that?*, lines 146–147) requesting information that the call-taker did not ask for. After receiving an answer to this question (*no, she is responsive, but with her thoughts, right?, she doesn't know?* lines 148–149), the interpreter turns back to the call-taker in Italian to report what she has collected from the caller (line 150, *allora*, *so*).

Nowhere in the call does the call-taker request the interpreter to ask if the patient's face shows any apparent sign of pain or distress. Among the actions available to an interpreter to solve comprehension problems are requests for clarification or requests for repetition (Baraldi & Gavioli, 2012). In the case briefly analysed here, the interpreter goes a step further: she does not ask the caller to clarify what she has just said. Instead, she introduces a brand-new question, as if she were the call-taker, not 'simply' an interpreter (Raymond, 2014b). Anticipating something that could possibly appear later in the talk, she appears oriented to the progressivity of the conversation. She tries to 'clarify the matter'—so to speak—by taking an autonomous initiative in the emergency, instead of simply acting on behalf of the call-taker. The interpreter thus shows that she is at the service of the activity, not merely of the call-taker.

5 Conclusion

As can be seen, when a linguistic problem arises in an emergency call, there are various possible solutions for the interactants, and the use of a professional interpreter is not the initial option: first, the caller, even when faced with an overt problem of comprehension, continues to speak in his/her language; then, a second person is reluctantly involved by the caller and the call-taker to act as an ad hoc mediator, if not as a real interpreter; finally, there is the possibility that a 'third mediating language' which pertains to neither the caller nor the call-taker can be used as a further communication resource.

Caller and call-taker can experience here a real linguistic barrier. If an ad hoc mediator cannot be found, or if there is no 'third language' that the parties can share, the risk is that the communication flow may be interrupted. The parties are confronted by the most severe kind of language problem, which may cause the complete collapse of communication. As we can see in the excerpts of this chapter, the definition itself of the problem's degree of severity and how it is addressed and managed are intrinsically bound up with, and negotiated in, the process of social interaction. The mere fact that the two people speak different languages and do not understand the language of the other does not in itself imply the existence of a language barrier. The diversity of languages can be an obstacle to communication in emergency calls, but it is only how this problem is dealt with by the parties that defines the severity of the problem. The severity of the problem that two different languages are spoken is configured as a linguistic barrier only when it cannot be solved. The constitution of the problem is closely related to how the parties recognize, manage, minimize or capitulate to the impossibility of communicating. In emergency calls, the recognition of this communication boundary or barrier is always accompanied by a set of communication strategies that, while recognizing a problem, at the same time provide its solution on an ad hoc and local basis.

Many studies have emphasised the role of a professional interpreter in healthcare services as the key resource to overcome language barriers. As Karliner et al. (2007, 750) say, "[i]t is likely that the improved utilization and clinical outcomes are mediated by the ability of professional interpreters to overcome health communication barriers. Professional interpreters, through their experience, training, and knowledge of both medical and lay terminology are better able to communicate patients' symptoms and questions to clinicians, and clinicians' rationale for treatment and explanations of proper use of therapy to patients." Or Bauer and Alegría (2010): "Use of professional interpreters may improve disclosure in patient-provider communications, referral to specialty care, and patient satisfaction." And Flores et al. (2012): "Evidence suggests that optimal communication, patient satisfaction, and outcomes and the fewest interpreter errors occur when LEP patients have access to trained professional interpreters or bilingual providers."

In this chapter, I have underlined that this may not be true in emergency medicine and particularly in the case of emergency calls: not because a professional interpreter is useless (quite the contrary!) but because of the restrictions of this communication event and the activities that it involves under critical time constraints. The use of professional interpreting services is often only the last resort. As has been convincingly shown by other studies (Osvaldsson et al., 2013; Raymond, 2014a, 2014b; Penn et al. 2017; Garcia, 2022), in emergency calls where the language of the caller is different from the language of the call-taker, there is a lot of interactional work where meaning is negotiated and intersubjectivity is secured. The message is that, if there are communication impairments, there are systematic and methodical ways to deal with the problems on the spot once they have appeared. Second, once a professional interpreter service is used, a researcher should seriously consider the overall work of a professional interpreter. Research on emergency communication should not focus on the work of rendering alone, as if interpreting consists 'only' of translating faithfully from one language to another, minimizing errors in comprehension (Flores et al., 2003, 2012); it should also examine how the communicative event is shaped and organized in a complex way by the contribution of a third party, the interpreter, who participates in the interaction principally to coordinate the meanings and the understandings.

References

Baraldi, C., & Gavioli, L. (2012). Introduction: Understanding coordination in interpreter-mediated interaction. In C. Baraldi & L. Gavioli (Eds.), *Coordinating participation in dialogue interpreting* (pp. 1–21). John Benjamins.

Bauer, A. M., & Alegría, M. (2010). Impact of patient language proficiency and interpreter service use on the quality of psychiatric care: A systematic review. *Psychiatric Services, 61*(8), 765–773.

Betz, E., & Deppermann, A. (2021). OKAY in responding and claiming understanding. In E. Betz, A. Deppermann, L. Mondada, & M.-L. Sorjonen (Eds.), *OKAY across languages: Toward a comparative approach to its use in talk-in-interaction* (pp. 55–92). John Benjamins.

Bradley, S. M., Fahrenbruch, C. E., Meischke, H., Allen, J., Bloomingdale, M., & Rea, T. D. (2011). Bystander CPR in out-of-hospital cardiac arrest: The role of limited English proficiency. *Resuscitation, 82*(6), 680–684.

Burke, P. (2006). The hybridization of languages in early modern Europe. *European Review, 14*(1), 105–110.

Carroll, L. N., Calhoun, R. E., Subido, C. C., Painter, I. S., & Meischke, H. W. (2013). Serving limited English proficient callers: A survey of 9-1-1 police telecommunicators. *Prehospital and Disaster Medicine, 28*(3), 286–291.

Cromdal, J. (2012). Conversation analysis and emergency calls. In C. Chapelle (Ed.), *The encyclopaedia of applied linguistics*. Wiley-Blackwell.

Emerson, R. M. (1981). On last resorts. *The American Journal of Sociology, 87*(1), 1–22.

Flores, G., Laws, M. B., Mayo, S. J., Zuckerman, B., Abreu, M., Medina, L., & Hardt, E. J. (2003). Errors in medical interpretation and their potential clinical consequences in paediatric encounters. *Pediatrics, 111*(1), 6–14.

Flores, G., Abreu, M., Barone, C. P., Bachur, R., & Lin, H. (2012). Errors of medical interpretation and their potential clinical consequences: A comparison of professional versus ad hoc versus no interpreters. *Annals of Emergency Medicine, 60*(5), 545–553.

Garcia, A. C. (2022). Interactional challenges for non-native speakers of English in emergency telephone calls. *Journal of Pragmatics, 193*, 222–234.

Gavioli, L. (2012). Minimal responses in interpreter-mediated medical talk. In C. Baraldi & L. Gavioli (Eds.), *Coordinating participation in dialogue interpreting* (pp. 201–249). John Benjamins Publishing.

Gavioli, L., & Baraldi, C. (2011). Interpreter-mediated interaction in healthcare and legal settings: Talk organization, context and the achievement of intercultural communication. *Interpreting, 13*(2), 205–233.

Gerwing, J., & Indseth, T. (2016). Enhancing caller comprehensibility in emergency calls with a language barrier: Operators in the role of addressee. *International Journal of Listening, 30*(3), 163–179.

Goffman, E. (1979). Footing. *Semiotica, 25*(1–2), 1–29.

Haffner, L. (1992). Translation is not enough. Interpreting in a medical setting. *Western Journal of Medicine, 157*(3), 255.

Heritage, J., & Clayman, S. E. (2010). Calls for emergency service. In J. Heritage & S. Clayman (Eds.), *Talk in action: Interactions, identities, and institutions* (pp. 53–100). Wiley-Blackwell.

Holt, E. (2017). Indirect reported speech in storytelling: Its position, design, and uses. *Research on Language and Social Interaction, 50*(2), 171–187.

Jacobs, E., Chen, A. H., Karliner, L. S., Agger-Gupta, N. I. E. L. S., & Mutha, S. (2006). The need for more research on language barriers in health care: A proposed research agenda. *The Milbank Quarterly, 84*(1), 111–133.

Kale, E., & Syed, H. R. (2010). Language barriers and the use of interpreters in the public health services. A questionnaire-based survey. *Patient Education and Counseling, 81*(2), 187–191.

Karliner, L. S., Jacobs, E. A., Chen, A. H., & Mutha, S. (2007). Do professional interpreters improve clinical care for patients with limited English proficiency? A systematic review of the literature. *Health Services Research, 42*(2), 727–754.

Meischke, H., Chavez, D., Bradley, S., Rea, T., & Eisenberg, M. (2010). Emergency communications with limited-English-proficiency populations. *Prehospital Emergency Care, 14*(2), 265–271.

Meischke, H. W., Calhoun, R. E., Yip, M. P., Tu, S. P., & Painter, I. S. (2013). The effect of language barriers on dispatching EMS response. *Prehospital Emergency Care, 17*(4), 475–480.

Mondada, L., & Sorjonen, M.-L. (2021). OKAY in closings and transitions. In E. Betz, A. Deppermann, L. Mondada, & M.-L. Sorjonen (Eds.), *OKAY across languages: Toward a comparative approach to its use in talk-in-interaction* (pp. 94–127). John Benjamins.

Ong, B. N., Yip, M. P., Feng, S., Calhoun, R., Meischke, H. W., & Tu, S. P. (2012). Barriers and facilitators to using 9-1-1 and emergency medical services in a limited English proficiency Chinese community. *Journal of Immigrant and Minority Health, 14*(2), 307–313.

Osvaldsson, K., Persson-Thunqvist, D., & Cromdal, J. (2013). Comprehension checks, clarifications, and corrections in an emergency call with a nonnative speaker of Swedish. *International Journal of Bilingualism, 17*(2), 205–220.

Penn, C., Koole, T., & Nattrass, R. (2017). When seconds count: A study of communication variables in the opening segment of emergency calls. *Journal of Health Psychology, 22*(10), 1256–1264.

Penn, C., Watermeyer, J., & Nattrass, R. (2017). Managing language mismatches in emergency calls. *Journal of Health Psychology, 22*(14), 1769–1779.

Rasmussen, G., Wagner, J., Luke, K. K., & Pavlidou, T. (2002). Language choice in international telephone conversations. In K.K. Luke & T-S. Pavlidou (Eds.), *Telephone calls: Unity and Diversity in Conversational Structure across Languages and Cultures* (pp. 111–131). John Benjamins.

Raymond, G. (2003). Grammar and social organization: Yes/no interrogatives and the structure of responding. *American Sociological Review, 68*, 939–967.

Raymond, C. W. (2014a). Negotiating entitlement to language: Calling 911 without English. *Language in Society, 43*(1), 33–59.

Raymond, C. W. (2014b). Epistemic brokering in the interpreter-mediated medical visit: Negotiating "patient's side" and "doctor's side" knowledge. *Research on Language and Social Interaction, 47*(4), 426–446.

Schegloff, E. A. (1987). Analyzing single episodes of interaction: An exercise in conversation analysis. *Social Psychology Quarterly, 50*(2), 101–114.

Stivers, T., & Robinson, J. D. (2006). A preference for progressivity in interaction. *Language in Society, 35*(3), 367–392.

Svennevig, J., Gerwing, J., Jensen, B. U., & Allison, M. (2019). Pre-empting understanding problems in L1/L2 conversations: Evidence of effectiveness from simulated emergency calls. *Applied Linguistics, 40*(2), 205–227.

Whalen, J., Zimmerman, D. H., & Whalen, M. (1988). When words fail: A single case analysis. *Social Problems, 35*(4), 335–362.

CHAPTER 7

Responses and Dispatch on the Radio

Abstract This chapter is different from the others in the book. It focuses not on features of calls between callers and call-takers, but on communication between operators in the emergency operation centre: in particular, it will focus on the ways in which dispatch of assistance is deployed. What happens after someone rings a public safety answering point for help? How is the emergency handled? How is the emergency service put into action? Prompt and competent intervention, and assessment of the gravity of the situation in a few crucial seconds: these are the quality standards that regulate the organization of emergency operations centres. In this chapter, I shall seek to show that a dispatch of assistance does not consist purely of information transfer; it is also the outcome of intense coordination work among the actors involved, both face to face and through the mediation of technological apparatus. The chapter examines not only the organization of the dispatch but also the tacit collaboration practices used by call-takers and dispatchers in a public safety answering point to share the information needed to dispatch the requisite resources to the site of an emergency.

Keywords TraDispatching • Radio communication • Collaboration between call-takers and dispatchers • Ecology of workspaces

G. Fele, *Emergency Communication*,
https://doi.org/10.1007/978-3-031-26239-5_7

1 The Collaborative Production of Responses and Dispatching on the Radio

Whalen and Zimmerman (2005) have emphasised that the management of incoming telephone calls to an operations centre requires complex work of listening and sense-making by those who share the same work ecology as that of the operator speaking on the telephone. This complex work evades official registration and is therefore not recorded on audio tapes. As Whalen and Zimmerman (2005, p. 310) write:

> Although it is typically the case that requests for help and emergency assistance are initiated by these phone calls, a great deal more is involved in the regular execution and production of 'calls' than the conversational exchanges. It turns out that for most emergency organizations, [...] the occasion of a 'call' is not at all coterminous with what transpires in talk on the telephone but rather is best described as an *ongoing and developing sequence of actions*, actions that may well be initiated in a phone conversation but have to then get systematically formed up, through the closely coordinated work of the organization's staff, into a certified organizational event—into a 'call'.

I intend to show that the management of even apparently simple radio communications between the personnel of an operations centre and the crew of an emergency vehicle on the ground requires intense collaborative work between persons physically co-present in a public safety answering point (PSAP). This work is one of the significant aspects of this type of work setting, and it is largely overlooked if consideration is only based on the audio recordings of communications. The chapter also seeks to show how the characteristics themselves of the communications technology used—the radio—make specific collaborative practices possible. Unlike calls by telephone, for example, incoming radio calls are heard not only by the person at the receiver but also by all those in the vicinity of the radio set: everyone within earshot can listen to the communication without the use of special devices (like the loudspeaker button on a telephone). This is an authentic kind of 'broadcast talk' (Luff & Heath, 2002; Tjora, 2004; Wong & Blandford, 2001, 2002). The audibility of incoming radio calls enables the other operators in the centre to easily overhear and monitor the ongoing activity, often while engaged in other tasks. The operators are able to judge the importance of the incoming call and act accordingly. The radio creates a sound environment that allows simultaneous courses of action by those present and facilitates co-participation in a specific task.

Various studies have examined the distinctive features of communication via radio. Simmons (1974) analysed radio communications between airline pilots and air traffic controllers. His particular concerns were to show firstly that radio communication exemplifies a specialized use of language, based on a restricted code, and secondly that the serial structure of turn-taking in radio communication is substantially different from that of ordinary conversation, a normal characteristic of which is the possibility that the speakers' turns overlap. Strevens (1984) analysed maritime radio communications. He too was interested in how the language used to speak on the radio is an example of the specialized use of language standardized into a specific variety: namely, 'Seaspeak'. Also, Sanders (2003) analysed maritime radio communications in order to determine how the technological characteristics of the radio constrained 'spontaneous' communication (overlaps between speakers, laughter). Mellinger (1992, 1994) analysed radio communications between paramedics at the scene of an accident, and personnel at the operations centre, viewing these communications as a practical example of the occupational culture of paramedics 'in action'. Luff and Heath (2002) studied the use of radio by personnel operating a rapid urban transport system. The aim of their study was to show how the participants organized their communication according to the constraints imposed by the technology. They highlighted in particular a curious asymmetry in participation rights whereby the personnel at the operations centre decided what incoming radio calls were to be accepted and initiated, and how this affected the formulation of the reason for the call. Szymanski et al. (2006) analysed the way in which mobile radios enable a remote state of incipient talk between friends: that is, the ways in which participants can initiate, engage, disengage and re-engage in a state of conversation-in-progress. Falzon (2009) studied the way in which communication between controllers in an air traffic control centre and pilots on airborne flights was organized through verbal interaction mediated by VHF radio technology. Rautiainen et al. (2022) have analysed radio exchanges as part of patrolling exercises in military observer training in which one party identifies and repairs troubles in the message when the other party explicitly requests a repetition (with "say again").

Notwithstanding the specific properties attributed to communication by radio, compared to the telephone, all these studies describe radio communication as involving two people at each end of the signal.[1] This chapter shows that a dispatch, as a kind of communication via radio, can be

[1] With the notable exception of the work by Rautiainen et al. (2022), where they observe that "Radiotelephony is inherently dyadic, but the parties may consist of more than one person".

considered the product of practices between two 'parties', where one of the parties is not necessarily a single physical person. At the PSAP studied, the radio was at the core of highly complex tacit collaboration practices carried out by call-takers and dispatchers.[2]

2 The Context

The data presented here consist of video recordings made in an Italian PSAP handling emergency calls to the 118 number—a dedicated number for health and other medical emergencies.[3] In my research, I collected 45 hours of video recordings during an ethnographic work that lasted six months in 2003.[4] I also collected the audio recordings of incoming and outgoing telephone calls and radio communications during the days and hours when the video recordings were made.

At the time when I made the video recordings the work of handling emergencies at the PSAP was organized around two 'boxes' or booths (#3 and #4) that received calls requesting assistance (see Fig. 7.1):

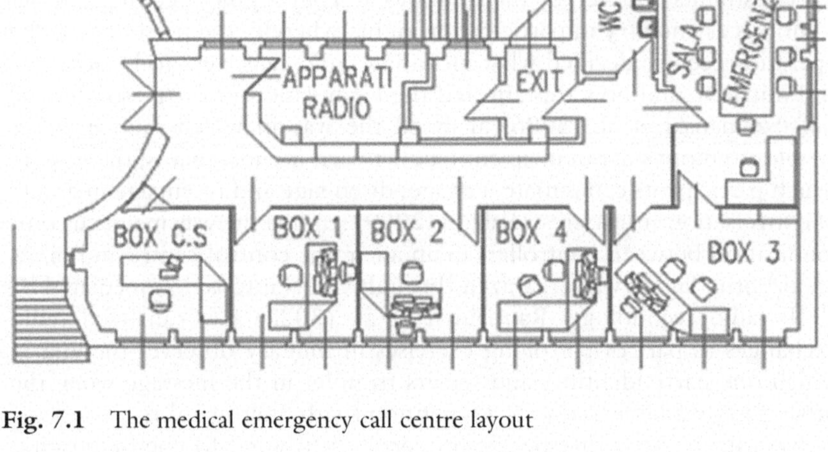

Fig. 7.1 The medical emergency call centre layout

[2] On the collaborative organization in the PSAP, see also Fele (2008, 2012).

[3] For the organization of a PSAP in Milan and Lombardy, see Gobo et al. (2008). For the Italian case, see also Dovigo and Redelli (2007, 2010) and Paoletti (2009).

[4] My presence at the PSAP continued intermittently in the following years, with other visits. I have been involved later in a project on teleambulance, on the exchange of video and images between ambulances on the scenes of emergencies and doctors and operators in the PSAP.

Box 3 and Box 4 dealt with calls coming from two different areas of the province. There was usually no communication between the two boxes because each of them handled emergencies independently and was self-sufficient. Although the workspace of each box was separate from the other, it was also permeable: it was possible to close the door and shut out interferences; but at the same time the walls were made of glass so that it was always possible at least to see what was going on in the other box.

Two operators worked side by side in each box.[5] They sat at a desk bearing computer screens, keyboards and mouses, radio sets, telephones, a closed-circuit television screen, sheets of paper, notebooks and so on (see Fig. 7.2):

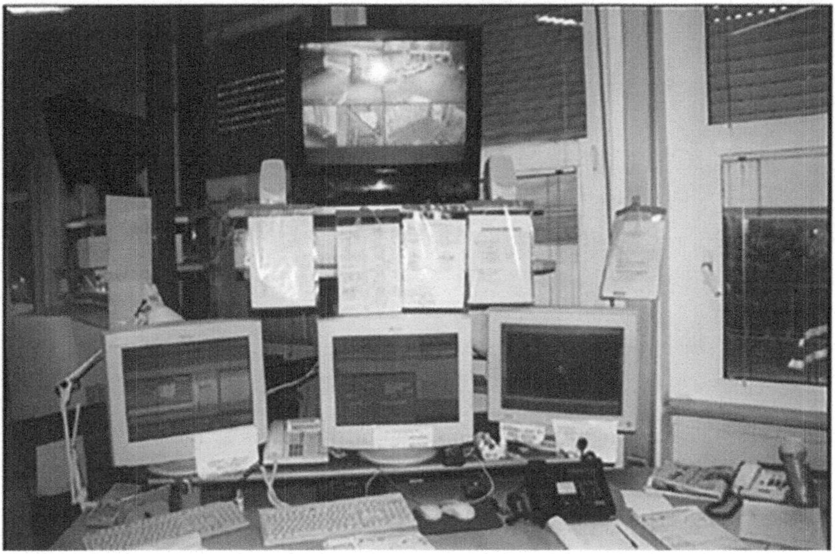

Fig. 7.2 The 'box' at the medical emergency call centre '118' at the time of the research

[5] This procedure is called 'horizontal' dispatching: that is, a tandem team approach to handling individual calls, compared to another procedure, called 'vertical' dispatching, "a method in which a single dispatcher handles all aspects of the call, including pre-arrival instructions, where necessary, as well as unit tone-out and en route information" (Clawson & Dernocoeur, 1988, p. 254).

A single emergency number—112—has now been implemented in the PSAP, following the European recommendations for a unique emergency number. This means that at the moment there are two PSAPs working: the PSAP1 where all the calls to a unique emergency number arrive; if a call is considered worthy of continuation, then the call is sent to three different PSAP2, depending on the kind of emergency.[6] The organization of the space has changed, and the organization of the work by the call-takers has changed accordingly. The division of labour between call-taker and dispatcher has remained more or less similar (Figs. 7.3 and 7.4).

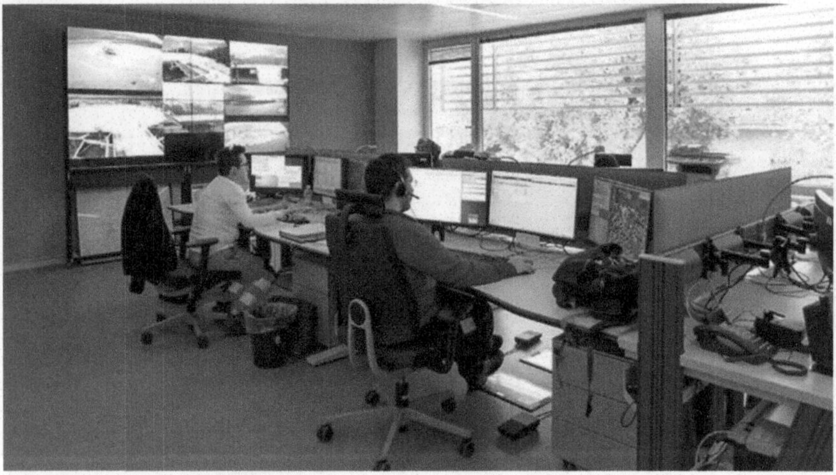

Fig. 7.3 The current (2022) organization of the spaces at the 112 emergency call centre. *Source*: https://www.ibtconnect.at/newseventi/

[6] The call arriving at the 112 unique emergency number can then be switched to the police call centre, to the ambulance call centre or to the firefighter call centre, depending on the kind of emergency. Kevoe-Feldman and Pomerantz (2018) analyse the procedure call-takers use to prepare callers for a transfer to a next call-taker.

[7] See Tjora (2000) on communicative between nurses and doctors in a Norwegian medical emergency call and dispatch centre.

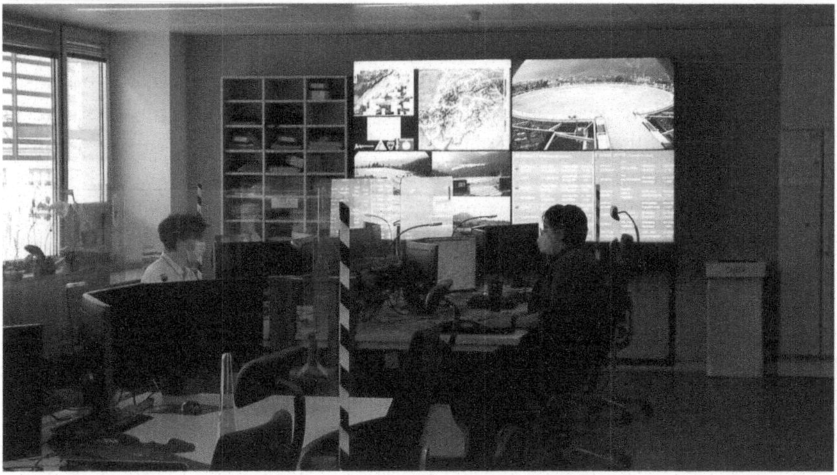

Fig. 7.4 The current (2022) organization of the spaces at the 112 emergency call centre. *Source*: https://www.ufficiostampa.provincia.tn.it/Comunicati/112-gestite-dalla-Centrale-Unica-di-Risposta-del-Trentino-200.000-chiamate-nel-2021

In the former organization of the dispatch centre that I analysed, calls to the dedicated number 118 were answered by two persons working together in a booth, with different institutional roles: one was in charge of answering the phone and receiving requests for assistance; the other was in charge of the dispatch. During their eight-hour work shift, these two persons more or less regularly alternated their roles, so that at one point the call-taker took over as dispatcher and vice versa. But this division of labour was not fixed once and for all, and it might happen, for instance, that the two operators dealt in parallel with two different incoming emergency calls: in these cases, each operator was dealing with one call and at the same time was in charge also of issuing the dispatch related to that call. There was in place a flexible organization of work that emerged in the course of events and which enabled the operators to manage contingent and unexpected aspects of their work. As Whalen and Zimmerman write, "what makes such teamwork possible is not only the structure and interdependency of institutional roles and responsibilities but the social relationships and interactional practices that develop among the participants over the course of *all* their conjoint activities" (Whalen & Zimmerman, 2005, p. 313).

When there were no screening of the incoming calls, there were many communicative activities going on at the PSAP 118: many incoming phone calls (a small number of which were emergency calls) from citizens but also from public authorities (like national and local police, firefighters, etc.); incoming radio calls, from ambulances and vehicles on the ground,[7] notifying where they were (at a hospital, at the site of an accident or back in the parking lot), or asking questions and seeking additional information; outgoing telephone and radio calls. In the case that I studied, the PSAP 118 was also in charge of sending ambulances to transfer patients from homes to hospitals, and vice versa. The PSAP 118 was usually a busy place, with numerous activities going on at the same time, often interconnected. Keeping track of all communicative activities would require a book in itself. Here I focus only on the activity of the first dispatch: that is, just after the call-taker has collected the necessary information from a call requesting help and reached a decision on sending a response (Hénault-Tessier & Dalle-Nazébi, 2012). The call-taker routes this information to the dispatcher, who contacts a specific unit for the response and transfers basic information so that an ambulance can immediately proceed to the site of the accident.

3 Radio Dispatch

Let us see in which ways these radio dispatches are organized. The first example concerns the dispatch of an emergency vehicle to assist a person stung by a wasp,[8] a radio communication between the dispatcher and a car ambulance. The following excerpt is taken from the official audio recording of the dispatch:

Excerpt 7.1 Dispatch 1. Wasp Sting

01 Dispat	attenzione cinque tre uno
	attention five three one
02 Radio	sì avanti
	yes go ahead

(*continued*)

[8] See in Chap. 4, Excerpt 4.4, the analysis of the beginning of the call requesting intervention related to this case.

Excerpt 7.1 (continued)

```
03 Dispat    andate in rosso
             proceed in red
04           in piazza Dante qui in città
             to Dante Square here in town
05           dove c'è il monumento,
             where the monument is
06           per una reazione anafilattica
             for an anaphylactic reaction
07           sembra grave.
             it seems severe.
08           guarda a:h,
             look a:h
09           si tratta di una vespa.
             it's a wasp.
10       (3.0)
11 Radio     occhei
             okay
```

The dispatch is organized according to what we can call a four-turn canonical procedure. The first turn is the summons ("attention five three one"), with which the dispatcher calls the attention of the crew of a specific ambulance (number 531). The ambulance crew responds to the summons ("yes go ahead"), making itself available to the service and authorizing the dispatcher to continue.[9] The dispatcher goes on to provide instructions: with an imperative verb ("proceed"), the dispatcher tells the ambulance where to go ("to Dante Square here in town, where the monument is"), with an emergency level code ("in red"[10]), with a formulation of the problem ("for an anaphylactic reaction") and an assessment of the situation ("it seems serious"). Here the dispatcher notifies also the cause of the problem, the anaphylactic reaction ("it's a wasp"). As soon as the

[9] Sometimes the ambulance crew is occupied with various activities, and it is not rare for the summons to be repeated.

[10] There are three levels of gravity, from the most severe situation (red) to the least (green), with an intermediate level (yellow).

dispatcher has finished transferring the 'information package' (Mellinger, 1992), all the critical information together in a cluster, the ambulance acknowledges its reception and moves into action. Each turn is accompanied by a unique possession of the communicative channel: in order to talk, the dispatcher presses a button, and releases it when she has finished. This is a signal for the other party to take the floor and talk. In this way, it is not possible for talk-turns to overlap. In terms of the turn design, there are no greetings and no personal identification. In addition, there is no other component of friendly talk like "how are you" and similar. I concur with what Rautiainen et al. (2022) said about this kind of communication: "Critical radio communication is pre-scripted and economical by nature. It has specific structural, lexical, and interactional features that clarify, simplify, and organise spoken interaction over distance" (69).

The second excerpt concerns a dispatch to a car accident on the motorway.[11]

Excerpt 7.2 Accident on the Motorway

```
01          ((buzzer not heard on the audio recording))
02 Radio    avanti, in ascolto.
            go ahead, you're on
03 Dispat   voi siete operativi cinque tre tre?
            are you operational five three three?
04 Radio    affermativo.
            affirmative.
05 Dispat   occhei, allora con infermiera, in rosso,
            okay, so with a nurse, on red,
06          in autostrada, direzione sud,
            on the motorway, southbound
07          (3.0)
08          al chilometro cento quaranta, uno quattro zero.
            at kilometre one hundred and forty, one four zero.
09          (3.0)
```

(*continued*)

[11] See in Chap. 4, Excerpt 4.3, the analysis of the beginning of the call requesting intervention related to this case.

Excerpt 7.2 (continued)

```
10 Ctaker   e::h nord e Ravina (.) cioè per arrivare (----)
            ((heard on the background))
            e::h North and Ravina (.) I mean, to arrive (---)
11 Dispat   tra Trento e Ravina, precisamente.=
            between Trento and Ravina, precisely=
12          =un ferito incosciente.
            an unconscious injured person.
13          entra anche l'auto medica.
            the medical car's coming as well.
14 Radio    bene.
            okay.
```

Here again, with few deviations, it is possible to identify the basic structure of a radio dispatch. The dispatcher pushes a button that activates a summons to the ambulance. The dispatcher begins an insertion sequence intended to determine if the selected ambulance (533) is on duty at that moment (*"are you operational five three three?"*). As soon as a member of the ambulance crew confirms that they are on duty (*"affirmative"*)—thus closing the inserted sequence—the dispatcher provides the "information package" (here the imperative verb is only implied), containing information regarding the composition of the ambulance crew ("with a nurse"),[12] the site of the accident ("on the motorway"), with instructions regarding where exactly on the motorway (that is also an instruction regarding the best route to take: "at kilometre one four zero, between Trento and Ravina, precisely"). Regarding the reason for the intervention, it is interesting that in this long turn there are no explicit references to "an accident", but only to what we can consider its aftermath ("an unconscious injured person"). This long turn is closed with the information that the ambulance will not be alone but that there will also be a medical car—that

[12] Only some of the ambulances have medical staff or nurses; the majority of interventions require only personnel able to stabilize the patient and send/her him to the nearest hospital or assistance hub, where the patient can receive—and only there—medical assistance. In general, the ambulance staff is composed of volunteers that have received specific training.

is, a dedicated car with a doctor—which is proceeding to the site of the accident. Once the information package has been completed, the dispatcher releases the button regulating access to the channel of communication. This again is the signal to the ambulance crew that the information is completed, and at this point a member of the crew confirms its reception ("okay").

To summarize, the dispatch can be said to consist of a four-turn sequence:

1. summons by the radio caller;
2. response by the operations centre, which authorizes the dispatcher to proceed;
3. the dispatcher provides the 'information package';
4. the operations centre acknowledges having received the information.

What is interesting to note at this point is that the dispatcher is the only authorized speaker on the radio. In this capacity, she is able to issue instructions to her interlocutor. In reality, however, what appears on the official surface of the transcript (and on the audio file) is only the final product of complex collective back-stage work between the two operators, call-taker and dispatcher, working collaboratively and cooperatively (Goodwin, 1995) inside the 'box'.

4 Forms of Collaboration

I shall now analyse aspects of the coordination and collaboration emerging from the interaction between the two operators working together in a booth that could be caught by a video recording. It usually happened that each operator—call-taker and dispatcher—did his/her work independently and in parallel with the other. But at some point, the work of the dispatcher intersected with that of the call-taker, and vice versa. By means of a video analysis, I shall concentrate on the two episodes transcribed above.

It should be stressed that this mostly tacit mutual awareness of what is happening between two operators sharing the same work space is omitted from the official documents. The official audio recordings of phone or radio communications retain few traces of the collaborative and participative work among the operators. Of course, the official audio recordings powerfully document collaboration and coordination between the people at the two ends of the telephone or radio line. What they do not document is the cooperation and collaboration that goes on among the people at each end of that line. Video recordings provide access to precisely that cooperation and collaboration (Heath & Luff, 2006; Heath et al., 2010; Mondada, 2006, 2008).[13] In order to analyse forms of multimodal collaboration[14] between the operators, it is necessary to leave the official audio recordings and examine what happened in the booth between the operators at that particular moment.[15]

4.1 "It's a Wasp"

If we consider the ecological context of the dispatch more broadly by analysing the organization of the work which enabled delivery of the dispatch, the definition of the dispatcher's work becomes more closely specified. The task of a dispatcher is not only to deliver information to an ambulance; it is also to obtain the relevant information to dispatch. This entails considering also the work of the call-taker in the booth and the ways in which dispatcher and call-taker work together to share the information available. Let us review the first case.

[13] For detailed examples and rich discussions on the use of video to document the practice of work in call centres, see Licoppe and Relieu (2005), Relieu et al. (2010) and Tuncer (2016). In particular, Rollet's PhD thesis (2012) is grounded on video recordings of the SAMU (*Service d'Aide Médicale Urgente*) operators answering to the emergency number "15" based in Versailles, France.

[14] On multimodality, see Mondada (2014, 2018, 2022).

[15] Kevoe-Feldman (2019, p. 238) urges researchers studying emergency call centres "to have more ethnographic information on the call centres that provides data, as having a members' understanding of the intricacies of the organizational constraints and processes can help make sense of the various contingencies that call-takers need to manage with their callers". I think that video analysis as a form of "focused ethnography" (Knoblauch, 2006; Knoblauch & Schnettler, 2012) makes it possible to untangle the intricacies and delicacies of these contingencies while conserving their details and preserving them for analysis. See Mondada (2006, 2008). See also Büscher (2005). For an outstanding dissertation using conversation analysis based on ethnographic fieldwork on a Swedish emergency call centre, see Hedman (2016). Rollet's dissertation (Rollet 2012) is based on audio-visual recordings collected at the Center of Reception and Regulation of Calls of the SAMU of Versailles (France). See also Tjora (2009).

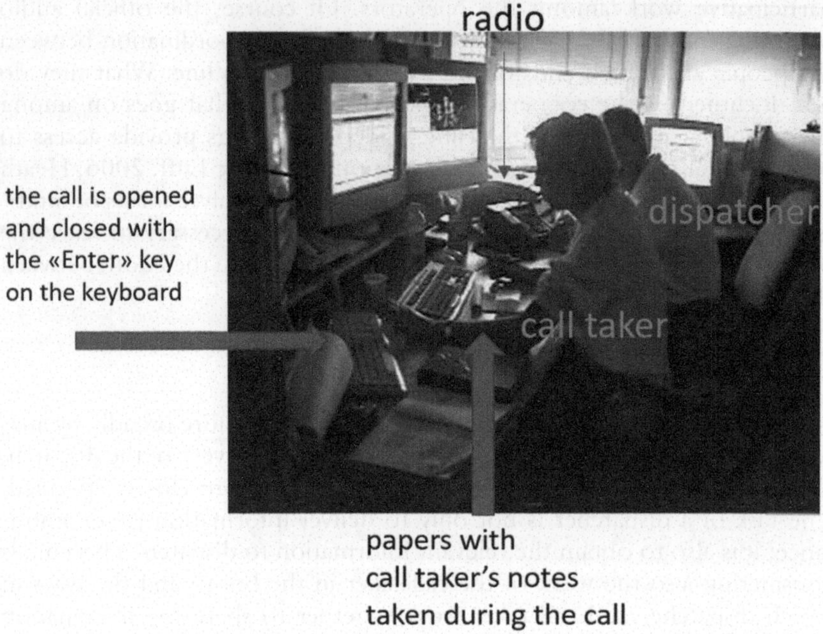
radio
the call is opened
and closed with
the «Enter» key
on the keyboard
dispatcher
call taker
papers with
call taker's notes
taken during the call

Fig. 7.5 Wasp sting: Call-taker and dispatcher working together in the booth

At the beginning of the episode, the call-taker is about to close the call where the caller was asking for help for a person stung by a wasp, and the dispatcher is looking at her (in Fig. 7.5, we can see his head turned to his left).

The following transcript requires some attention. I have tried to render the sequential organization of three different dyadic interactions as they developed over time with their natural mutual swapping and overlapping: the first interaction is between the caller and the call-taker; the second is between the call-taker and the dispatcher; the third is between the dispatcher and the emergency unit (the actual dispatch is in bold).

Excerpt 7.3 Wasp Sting—Video Dispatch (Duration: 18 Sec.)

```
01 Ctaker   d'accordo? ((closing the phone call))
            okay?
02          saluti, arrive[de(rci)    ]
            bye, see you
03 Dispat                     [gli mandiam] l'auto medica?
            ((to the call-taker))
                               shall we send the ambulance car?
04 Ctaker   sì, in [          rosso:::          ]
            yes, in            red
05 Dispat          [attenzione cinque tre uno]
                    attention five three one
06 Ctaker   (è andà su-), sì,
            (he's going up-), yes,
07          intanto l'auto medica, dai. in [piazza Dante,=
            meanwhile the ambulance car, yes. in Dante Square,=
08 Radio                                   [sì  avanti   ]
                                             yes go ahead
09 Ctaker   =>proprio vicino al mo[numento,<    ]
            =>right near to the monument<
10 Dispat                             [andate in rosso]
                                       proceed in red
11          in piazza Dante qui in città
            to Dante Square here in town
12          dove c'è il monumento↑,
            where the monument is,
13 Ctaker   per una reazione ana[filattica::,=
            for an anaphylactic reaction::,=
14 Dispat                        [per una reazione anafilattica:
                                  for an anaphylactic reaction
15 Ctaker   =sembra [grave
            =apparently severe
16 Dispat           [sembra grave.
                     apparently severe.
14          (.)
```

(*continued*)

Excerpt 7.3 (continued)

15		**guarda a:h, si tratta di una vespa**
		look a:h, it's a wasp
17	Ctaker	hhhhhhhhhhh ((laughing))
18		h h h
19		il paziente è una vespa
		the patient is a wasp ((laughing))
20		°hhhhh hhh °hhhh h h h
21		"il eh- sembra grave", la vespa è grave
		"the eh- is seriously ill", the wasp is ill
22		°hhhh
23	Dispat	senti, gli mando incontro la:,
		listen, I'll send after him the
24		la [( ) anche]
		the (----------) also
25	Ctaker	[manda la cinque] quattro otto
		send the five four eight
26		[sì
		yes:,
27	**Radio**	**[occhei**
		okay

The call-taker is completing the telephone call requesting an ambulance to treat a wasp sting (lines 1 and 2). The dispatcher has already positioned his hands near to the radio set, in particular on the button that is used to open the communication channel (see Fig. 7.6).

The dispatcher addresses his colleague before she has completed both the telephone call and her turn (note the overlap between the call-taker's turn at line 2 and the dispatcher's turn at line 3). The dispatcher has heard the telephone call, but he does not have access to the information that the caller has given to the call-taker (the call-taker is wearing earphones). He has heard only what the call-taker repeated aloud during the conversation. As well known in the literature on workplace studies (Luff et al., 2000; Goodwin & Goodwin, 1996), this is a formidable source of orientation for all those present in the setting, in that a colleague's repetitions aloud and his/her questions make publicly available—'on air' so to speak—salient elements of the communication which may have procedurally

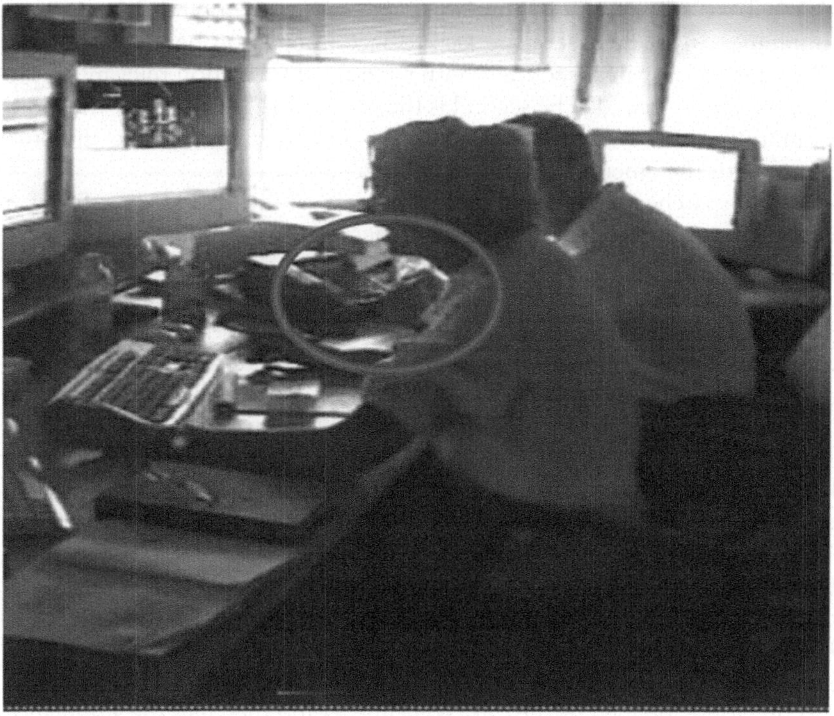

Fig. 7.6 The focus is on the finger on the radio button

important consequences for the subsequent actions of other colleagues. I point out that the dispatcher is able to anticipate the next relevant action (sending an ambulance) without being given any explicit instructions. The dispatcher's turn is designed as a proposal in interrogative form (line 3: "shall we send the ambulance car?"): that is, his turn projects a pertinent action by his colleague which consists in confirming or disconfirming the proposal. The call-taker, who has just ended the telephone call, immediately answers her colleague. She agrees with his proposal (line 4, "yes", means "I confirm that in this case the ambulance car should be sent") and adds another crucial element to the dispatch delivery, namely the urgency of the event. In this case, the gravity of the incident is indicated by its being flagged as "red" (line 4: "yes, in red"). The operation code must now be communicated to the crew of the ambulance car.

What we see in action now are two systems of interaction working simultaneously. The first is the face-to-face interaction between the call-taker and the dispatcher in the booth whereby information relevant to the intervention is shared. The second is the interaction mediated by the radio communications system which connects the dispatcher in the dispatch centre with the emergency crews on the ground.

The dispatcher contacts an ambulance car (number 531, line 5) even before the call-taker has completed her turn.[16] The communication between the call-taker and the dispatcher proceeds in parallel with the communication between the dispatcher and the medical car crew. The call-taker sequentially produces item by item the information needed by the dispatcher to deliver the dispatch. The dispatcher merely relays, almost automatically, the information as he receives it from the call-taker. The latter tells the dispatcher where the incident has occurred (line 8: *In Dante Square, right near to the monument*), which is the place where the ambulance car should head, sharing the information that she has jotted down on a piece of paper in front of her (see Fig. 7.7).

In the dispatcher's hands (or better his voice), this information furnished by the call-taker becomes an instruction issued to the ambulance car. The dispatcher resumes radio communication with the ambulance car even before the call-taker has completed her turn. The dispatcher begins the dispatch by stating the urgency code of the incident (line 10: *proceed in red*) as just previously defined by the call-taker (line 4) and then tells the ambulance car where it should go (lines 11–12: *to Dante Square here in town, where the monument is*) as the call-taker has described it in her immediately previous turn. At this point, the dispatcher's turn addressed to the ambulance car crew is suspended.[17] The call-taker has shifted her attention from her colleague to the computer screen in front of her. She is now logging the incident data in the call centre database (see Fig. 7.8).

At this perceived suspension,[18] although the call-taker does not interrupt her task (completing the computer form) or change her posture (she

[16] As we have observed, this turn corresponds to a summons, like the ringing of the telephone, but more individualized in the sense that identifies the receiver.

[17] It is difficult to ascertain in the video if the dispatcher lifts his finger or hand from the radio button, interrupting the information flow via the radio, but it is more than likely.

[18] I call it a 'perceived perception' because the dispatch is clearly not concluded. The items in the dispatch consist of the urgency code for the incident, and the place where it has occurred, and therefore where the ambulance car should go. One item is obviously still missing, that is, the type of incident: thus, discernible here is a suspension of the activity, which is also connected with the prosody of the dispatcher's turn. That this is a suspension perceived not by the analyst but by the actors themselves is evident from the rest of the interaction.

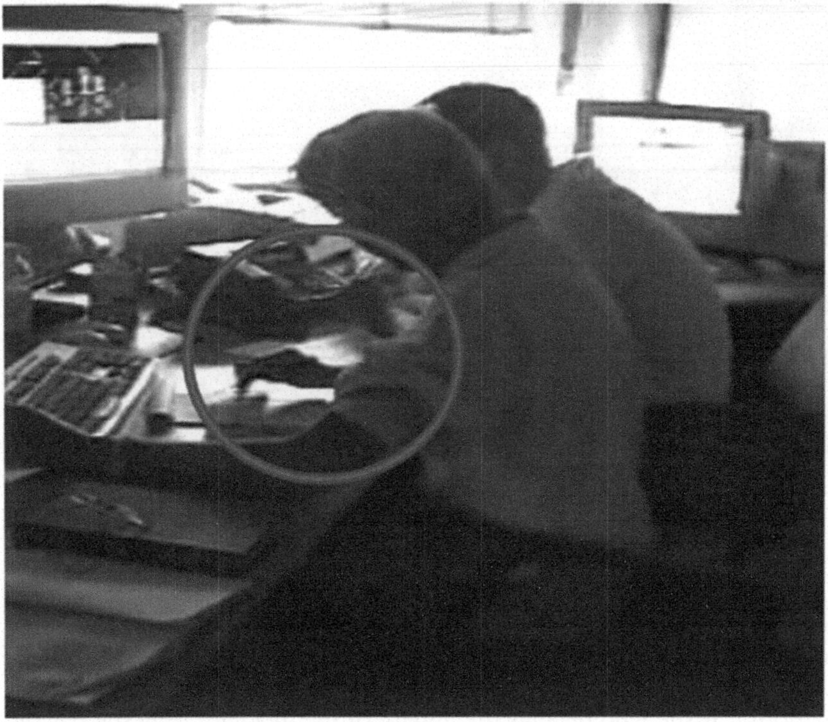

Fig. 7.7 The call-taker shows her notes to the dispatcher

is facing the computer screen with her hands on the keyboard—see Fig. 7.8), she provides her colleague with the information that he requires (line 13: *For an anaphylactic reaction, apparently severe*). Before the call-taker's turn has ended, the dispatcher resumes the communication via radio and repeats word-by-word the information that the call-taker has just given him (line 15: *For an anaphylactic reaction, apparently severe*). The dispatch is completed with a description of the cause of the anaphylactic reaction (line 15: *look a:h, it's a wasp*). This information elicits the call-taker's jocular aside that the dispatcher has formulated the information so that it seems that the victim is a wasp (lines 17–22).

If we consider this extract from the point of view of the actors' individual actions—and therefore consider each actor individually in terms of his/her ability to control his/her behaviour, the way in which his/her

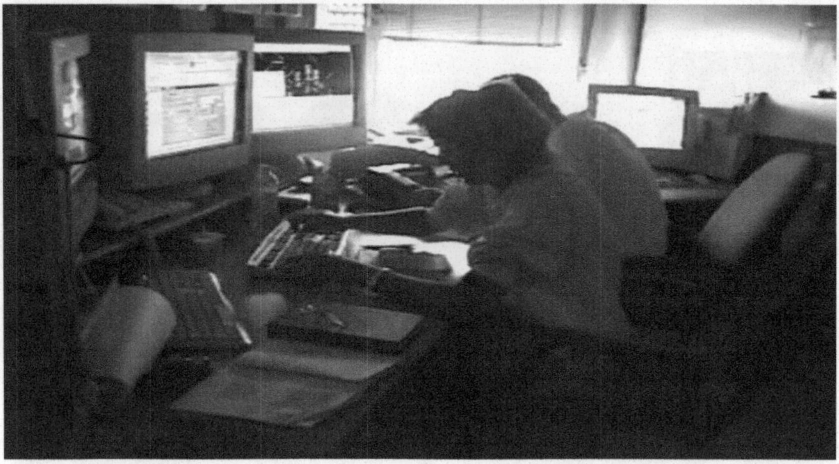

Fig. 7.8 The call-taker logs the incident data in the call centre database

actions have consequences for other actors, and possible assessment of the action performed—there seems to be an evident asymmetry of knowledge, power and control. The dispatcher resembles a simple 'sounding box' which repeats item-by-item over the radio the information provided by the call-taker.[19] Only the call-taker appears to be the repository of information: it is she who decides the gravity of the incident; only she has the relevant information; she is the author of the dispatcher's communication; and she is responsible for it. The dispatcher seemingly acts only as a 'ventriloquist's dummy'.

However, matters change if we examine the extract in terms of the interaction system. Just as an examination of the official audio recording of the dispatch (the transcript of the radio communication alone) does not bring out the collective collaboration which makes the work at the emergency call-centre possible, so an approach centred exclusively on individual action fails to grasp how the interaction system works. Only by analysing the situation as a whole is it possible to appreciate the subtle coordination work performed by physically co-present actors engaged in a common task. From this point of view, it does not make a great deal of sense to talk of an actor's greater or lesser freedom of action unless

[19] Goffman (1979) says that the speaker in a sense of a 'sounding box' "can share this physical function with a loudspeaker system or a telephone" (p. 17).

consideration is made of the constant work of reciprocal adjustment performed by the participants in order to anticipate each other's relevant actions and possible future moves. The dispatcher's initial turn (at line 5) begins before the end of the call where his colleague is collecting information about the case. The design of the turn shows that the dispatcher anticipates alternative actions possible at this point (line 3: *shall we send the ambulance car?*)—his question is not designed as a generic question (like, for instance, *what can we do now?*). Coordination between the parties assumes a markedly temporal and sequential character, especially when the dispatcher has launched the radio communication. The call-taker furnishes the items required by the dispatcher (the seriousness of the incident; where it has occurred; what has happened) in positions immediately antecedent to their relevance for the dispatch—that is, the work being performed by the dispatcher on the radio (Fig. 7.9).

The call-taker's information items are sequentially positioned: if the dispatch sent to the rescue team is packaged into a single communication format and reaches the end of the channel as a unit, the dispatch itself is built step-by-step by call-taker and dispatcher. The call-taker subtly guides the dispatcher by slightly anticipating the information content, positioning it at

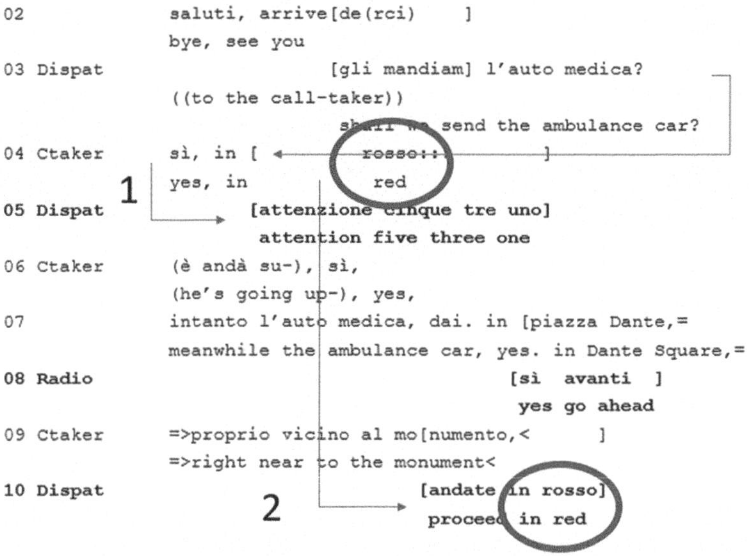

Fig. 7.9 Wasp sting: The organization of the dispatch—first part

the appropriate point and waiting for the next slot in which to insert the next item of information. The dispatcher for his part systematically anticipates his colleague's turn in order to speak on the radio, thereby establishing the rhythm of the face-to-face interaction. At the same time, the dispatcher elicits further information from the call-taker by stopping at the appropriate point, thereby orienting her attention and obtaining the further information. The intonation pattern of the dispatcher's turn (rising tone, line 12) indicates to the call-taker that the dispatch has not been completed and that a further item of information is required (Fig. 7.10).

All this takes place within the time frame of the ongoing emergency event. Hence, every decision about what to do and how to do it is compressed: the resources must be dispatched as soon as possible; knowing what to do must be almost entirely co-extensive with its being done. The transfer of relevant information from the call-taker (the informant) to the dispatcher (the informee) does not precede the phase when the dispatcher issues instructions to the ambulance car crew. The information is not first 'received' and then 'codified' and transformed into instructions. The process takes place *almost* instantaneously. It is fluid and efficient: no pause or interruption breaks the flow of the collective action. The outcome is a complex and interconnected system of professional practices produced within an important temporal constraint, where the temporal dimension is both 'external' to the interaction (the event's nature as an *emergency*) and internal to it.

```
07          intanto l'auto medica, dai. in [piazza Dante,=
            meanwhile the ambulance car, yes. in Dante Square,=
08 Radio                                   [sì  avanti  ]              3
                                            yes go ahead
09 Ctaker   =>proprio vicino al mo[numento,<        ]
            =>right near to the monument<
10 Dispat                             [andate in rosso]
                                       proceed in red
11          in piazza Dante qui in città
            to Dante Square here in town                  4
12          dove c'è il monumento↑,
            where the monument is,
13 Ctaker   per una reazione ana[filattica::,=
            for an anaphylactic reaction::,=
14 Dispat                        [per una reazione anafilattica:       5
                                  for an anaphylactic reaction
15 Ctaker   =sembra [grave
            =apparently severe
16 Dispat         [sembra grave.                    6
                   apparently severe.
```

Fig. 7.10 Wasp sting: The organization of the dispatch—second part

These are some aspects that an approach centred only on individual action seems unable to grasp.

4.2 *"Are You Operational 533?"*

Episodes like the one just described illustrate a common way in which dispatching was organized in the call centre that I studied. I now return to the second case.

I consider again what happens in the call-centre booth when the dispatch is delivered (Fig. 7.11).

The call-taker is about to finish talking to an operator at the motorway operations centre (denoted in the transcript as A22) about an apparent multi-car accident. What has actually happened is not yet clear—the caller was able to describe only that "there has been an accident",[20] but the machinery of the operations centre is already in motion. The call-taker is going to end her

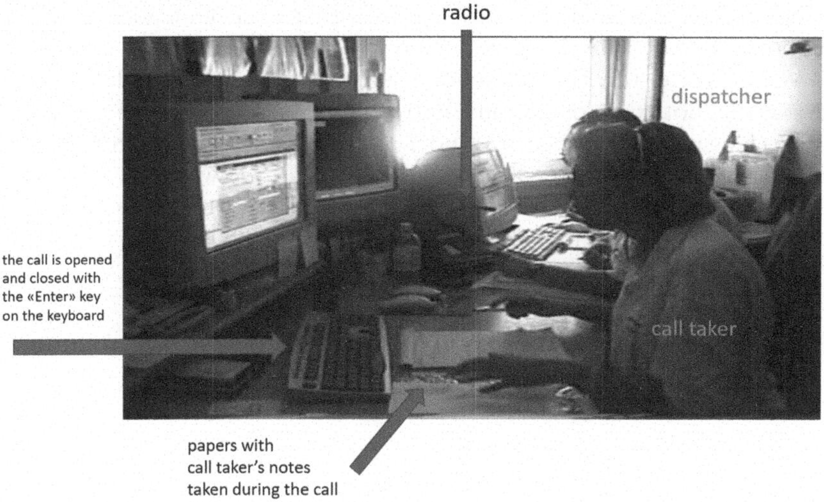
radio
dispatcher
the call is opened and closed with the «Enter» key on the keyboard
call taker
papers with call taker's notes taken during the call

Fig. 7.11 Accident on the motorway: The call-taker and the dispatcher working in the booth

[20] The caller was heading in the opposite direction to the accident. Hence, from her car she was able to see only briefly what had happened on the other carriageway. See Chap. 4, Excerpt 4.3.

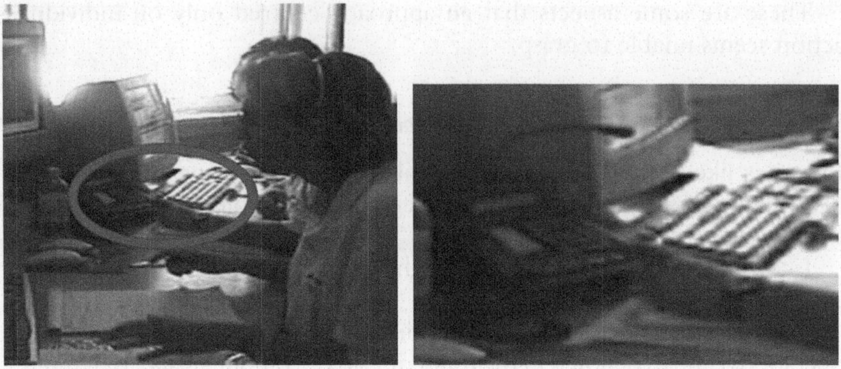

Fig. 7.12 **a, b** The dispatcher ready to issue a communication via radio (and detail)

call when the dispatcher has called an ambulance crew by radio—this time by using a button on the radio console, not with a vocal summons (as in the previous extract)—and is waiting for a response (Fig. 7.12).

While the call-taker is ending her telephone conversation with the operator at the motorway operations centre, the response arrives on the radio.

Here again I have tried to render the sequential organization of the interaction between the caller and the call-taker, between the call-taker and the dispatcher and between the dispatcher and the emergency unit (the actual dispatch is in bold).

Excerpt 7.4 Accident on the Motorway—Video *Dispatch*[21]

```
07 Ctaker   #va beh, comunque intanto
            okay, anyway meanwhile
                 #figure
08          io mando. d'accordo?
            I'll send. okay?
09 A22      centoquaranta sud, allo[ra.
            one hundred forty South, then
```

(*continued*)

[21] I have indicated overlaps between speakers officially engaged in a conversation with the sign "[". I have indicated overlaps between speakers not officially engaged together in a conversation with the sign "*".

Excerpt 7.4 (continued)

```
10 Ctaker                                   [va *benissimo.*
                                             it's very good
11 Radio                                      *avanti, in ascol*to.
                                               go ahead, you're on.
12 A22        proprio all'altezza di Ravina.
              just right at Ravina
13 Dispat     voi siete o*perativi cinque tre tre?
              are you operational five three three?
14 Ctaker              *perfetto, grazie.
                        perfect, thanks.
16 Radio      affermativo.
              affirmative.
17 Dispat     occhei,
              okay
18            allora con l'infermiera,
              so, with a nurse
19            in rosso, in autostrada,
              on red, on the motorway,
20            direzione sud,
              southbound direction
21      -->   dove? ((to the call-taker))
              where?
22 Ctaker     allora, al chilometro centoquaranta.
              well, at kilometre one hundred and forty.
23 Dispat     al chilometro cento quaranta,
              at kilometre one hundred and forty,
24            uno quattro zero.
              one four zero.
25      -->   sai mica a cosa corrisponde. ((to the call-taker))
              do you know what it corresponds to.
26 Ctaker     eh, tra Trento:: nord e Ravina.
              eh, between Trento::: North and Ravina.
27            (cioè), nei pressi di-,
              (that is), near-
28            cioè per arrivare a *Ravi-.
              I mean to arrive at Ravi-
```

(continued)

Excerpt 7.4 (continued)

```
29 Dispat                          *tra Trento e Ravina,
                                    between Trento and Ravina,
30          pre*cisamente.
            precisely.
31 Ctaker      *esatto.
                right.
32 Dispat   un ferito incosciente.
            an unconscious injured person.
33          entra anche l'auto medica.
            the ambulance car's coming as well.
34 Ctaker   non so, siccome che, l'autostrada
            I don't know, because at the motorway
35          non aveva notizie precise
            they didn't have precise information
36 Radio    bene.
            good.
```

The call-taker is talking on the telephone to the operator at the motorway operations centre[22]: although unsure as to what has happened, she is communicating that she will send an ambulance to the scene of the supposed accident (lines 7–8: *okay, anyway meanwhile I'll send. Okay*?). The motorway operator repeats to the call-taker the coordinates of the supposed scene of the accident (line 9: *one hundred forty South, then*—that is, kilometre 140 on the southbound carriageway) and then immediately adds a less technical description of the location of the accident (line 12: *just right at Ravina*—a small town adjacent to the motorway). The telephone call now ends with the call-taker's acknowledgement turn (line 14: *perfect, thanks*).[23] The closure of the telephone call overlaps with the beginning of the radio communication between the dispatcher and the ambulance. These are two independent courses of action which proceed in parallel.

[22] Remember that the call-taker is using headphones, so only what the call-taker says aloud is audible also to the dispatcher. Here I have transcribed the end of the audio file of the telephone call that I retrieved and saved from the information system the day after this video recording.

[23] The call ends here in a rather abrupt way, where the motorway operations centre does not provide any closing item or greeting in return.

The dispatcher, after having pressed the radio button (the "buzzer") to call the ambulance crew, moves closer to her a notepad on which the call-taker has jotted down some information regarding the event in order to read it. In this way, she is again anticipating the vocal transfer of information that the call-taker is going to perform after closing the call with the motorway operations centre. See first how the call-taker raises her right elbow to facilitate the dispatcher's access to the notes, and then how both of them look at the notes (Figs. 7.13 and 7.14):

After receiving the signal that the radio channel is open (line 11: *go ahead, you're on*), the dispatcher also obtains the operational availability of the ambulance called (line 13 *are you operational five three three*, where '533' is the vehicle identification number; the crew answers in the affirmative—line 16). The dispatcher is oriented with her face towards the colleague, not towards the radio—this is the best way to be attuned to whatever new information may come from her colleague (Fig. 7.15), who is about to close the call and is shifting her arms so that she can reach the computer keyboard and log the information regarding the accident.

Having assured the availability of the ambulance, the dispatcher begins the delivery of the dispatch by furnishing a series of initial items of information: the composition of the ambulance crew, the incident urgency code and a first formulation of the place of the accident (lines 18–20: *so,*

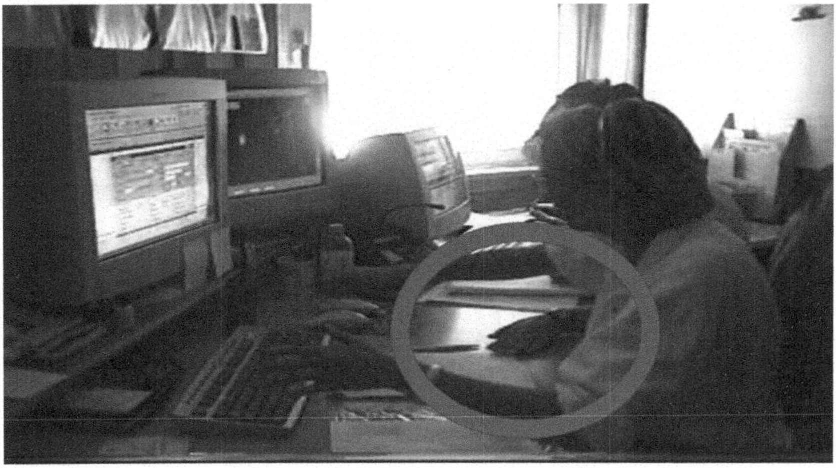

Fig. 7.13 The dispatcher reaches the call-taker's notes with her left hand

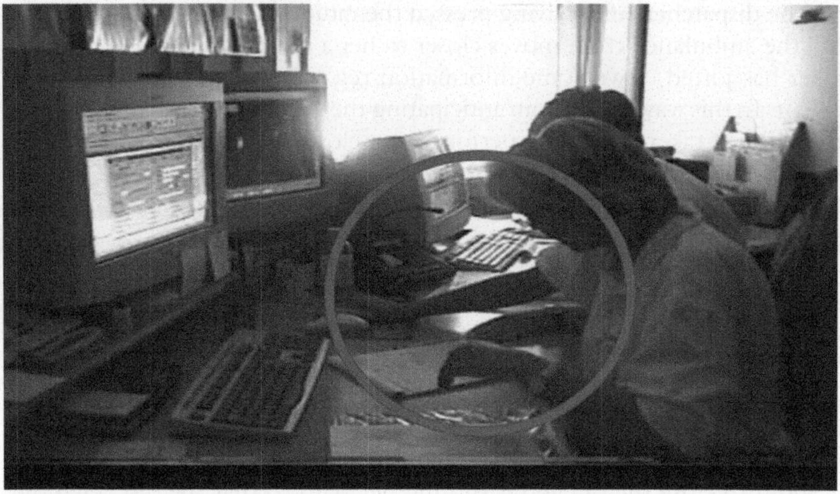

Fig. 7.14 The call-taker raises her arm in order to facilitate the reading of the notes by the dispatcher

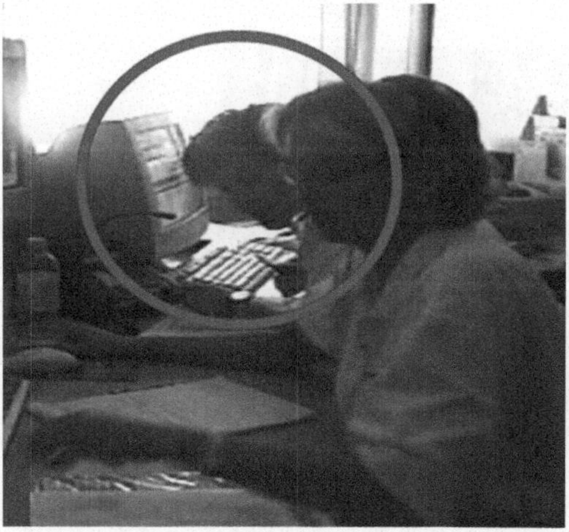

Fig. 7.15 The dispatcher talks on the radio while at the same time being oriented towards her colleague

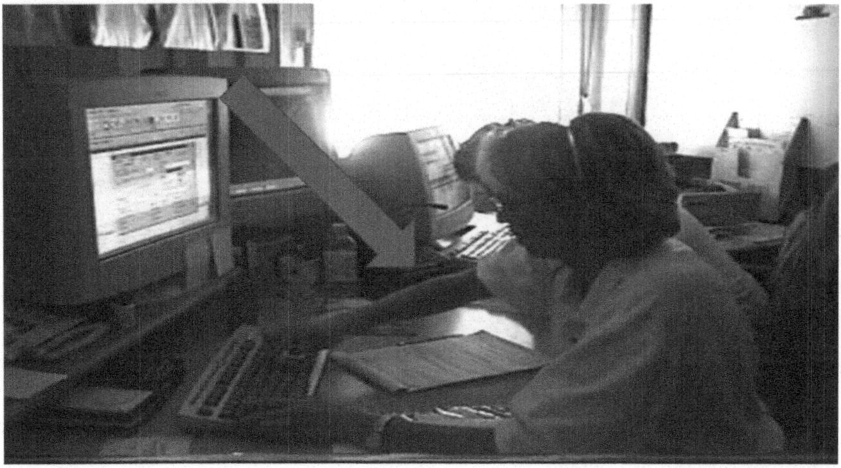

Fig. 7.16 The call-taker helps the dispatcher read her notes by raising her right arm

with a nurse, on red, on the motorway, southbound). The dispatcher is able to have visual access to the call-taker's notes also because the call-taker slightly raises her right arm when using the keyboard. See Fig. 7.16:

Just before stating on the radio the location of the accident (line 19 "on the motorway"), the dispatcher uses her left arm (her right hand is continuing to push the button opening the radio communication channel) to move the notepad towards her (Fig. 7.17a) so that she can read its content to the ambulance crew. The call-taker momentarily suspends her logging activities and with a rapid pointing movement (Fig. 7.17b) indicates to the dispatcher where she has jotted down the location ("direction South bound", line 20). Then she returns to her previous tasks:

At this point, the dispatcher lifts her finger from the button which, when pressed, keeps the radio link open, and asks her colleague for further information about the location of the accident (line 21: *where?*). The communication is addressed solely to her colleague: nothing of it is recorded in the official transcript of the radio conversation. The call-taker answers her colleague's question by giving further information obtained from the motorway operations centre (line 22: *so, at kilometre one hundred and forty*).

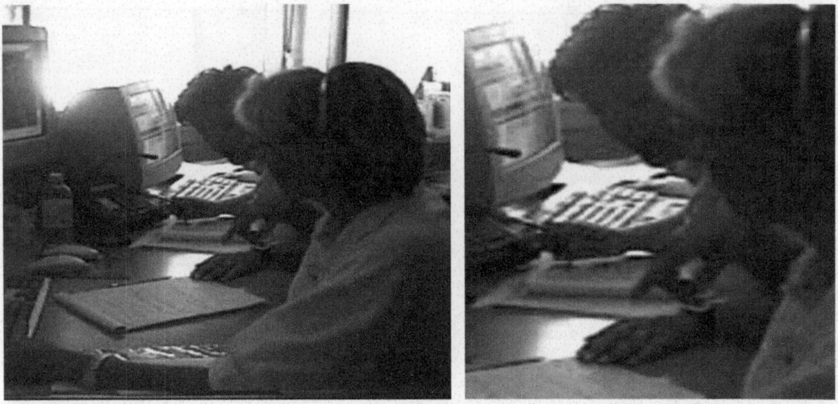

Fig. 7.17 **a** and **b** The call-taker points to her notes while being oriented to her computer screen (and detail)

At this point, the call-taker completely leaves her position in front of the computer screen and turns to the written notes, not only telling the information to the dispatcher but also pointing firmly at the written source—see Fig. 7.18:

When the call-taker returns to her computer task, the dispatcher immediately resumes the communication via radio (by once again pressing the button to open the channel) and repeats to the ambulance crew the information just obtained from her colleague (lines 23–24: *at kilometre one hundred and forty, one four zero*). The dispatcher again interrupts the radio communication (by lifting her finger from the button and closing the channel) to ask her colleague for further information (line 25: *do you know what it corresponds to*—Fig. 7.19). Neither is this communication recorded by the official transcript. The call-taker answers by providing further information with which to identify the exact place of the accident (lines 26–28: *between Trento:: North and Ravina. (that is), near- I mean to arrive at Ravi-*).

This information is relayed by the dispatcher on the radio in her immediately following turn (lines 29–30: *between Trento and Ravina, precisely*), while still being oriented toward her colleague (Fig. 7.20).[24] The colleague confirms (line 31: *right*).

[24] Interestingly, the second description of the place (*between Trento and Ravina, precisely*) is given with 'precision'. Apparently, the first formulation (*at kilometer one hundred and forty, southbound)* should have been more 'objective' and therefore more precise.

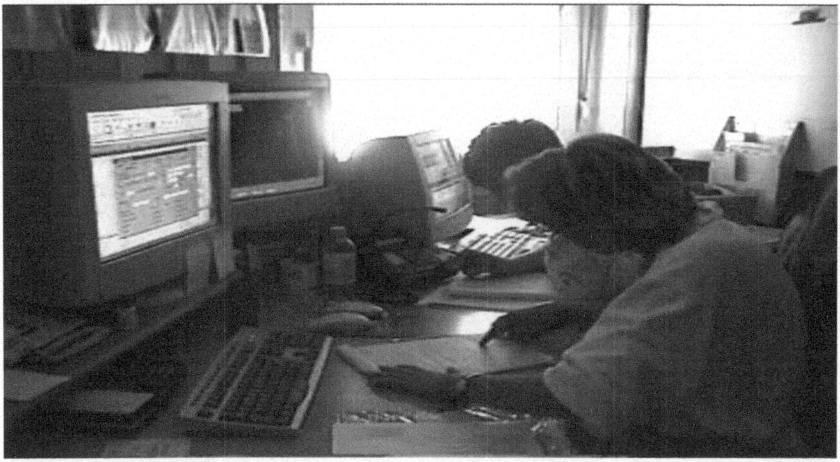

Fig. 7.18 The call-taker points to the dispatcher the relevant information in her notes

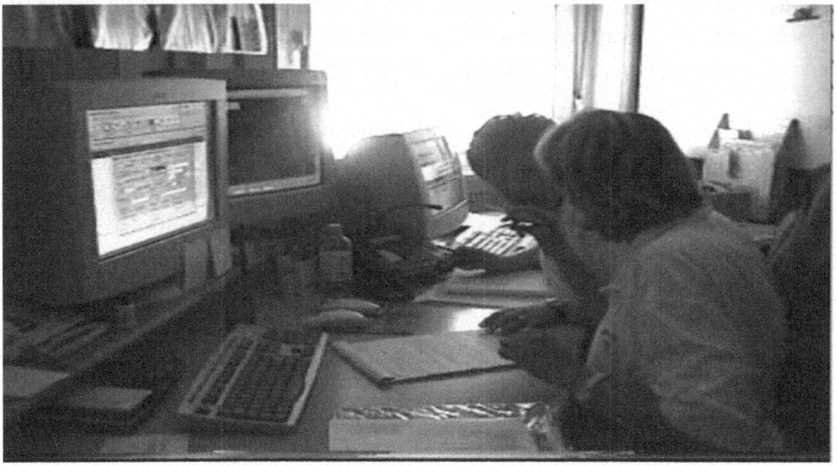

Fig. 7.19 The dispatcher addresses her colleague regarding the location of the incident

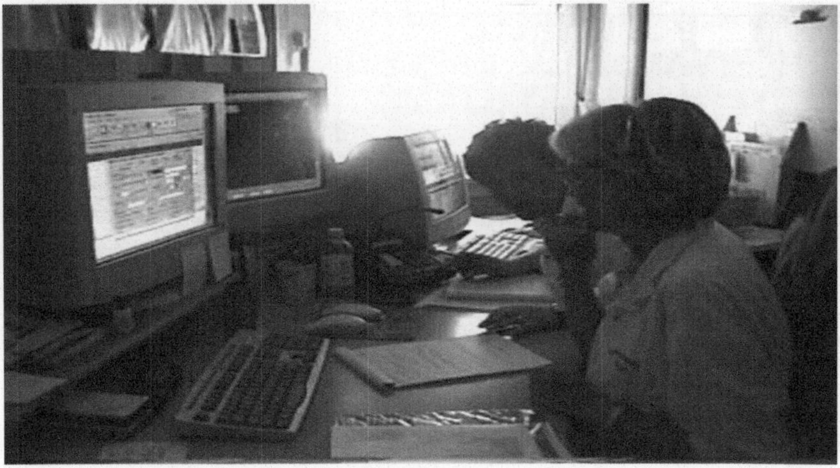

Fig. 7.20 The dispatcher talks on the radio while at the same time continuing to look at her colleague

The dispatcher proceeds with the dispatch, furnishing the final items of information of relevance to the event (lines 32–33: *an unconscious injured person. the ambulance car's coming as well*). Then the radio confirms reception (line 36: *good*).

The entire episode lasted about 30 seconds. What I have described at length happened at great speed. The dispatcher alternated her participation between two regimes: that of physical proximity, or the face-to-face interaction with her colleague; and that of mediated communication with the ambulance crew. This alternation enabled her to operate in a situation with a temporal imperative to act rapidly, to anticipate events and to accelerate responses to an emergency. But at the same time, the dispatcher did not have sufficient information or a complete picture of the situation. The dispatcher thus initiated a course of action by opening the radio communication and sending the dispatch at the same time as she was simultaneously acquiring the information. The dispatcher's knowledge in regard to the ongoing event was therefore not a prerequisite for communication. The amount of information in possession of the dispatcher increased as the interaction with the call-taker proceeded. The dispatcher's transition from lack of information to knowledge resulted from cooperative work and subtle coordination with the colleague sitting beside her precisely as she was pursuing an independent course of action. In cases like this, concentrating on the properties of a single individual does not make it possible to grasp the emergent characteristics generated by an entire system of interaction. On examining the organization of the interaction, it is possible to appreciate that the skills exhibited by the dispatcher on the radio (as they emerge from the official audio recording) were nothing other than the products of intense collective concertation work which produced competence as the final outcome of, not the prerequisite for, communication.

5 Conclusions

The chapter has shown how the operators at a call centre handling medical emergencies tacitly collaborated in managing radio communications with the crew of a vehicle on the ground.

It is interesting to see how this activity was distributed. Video recordings of ongoing activity in the booth give access to the work performed by the two parties in tacitly or openly distributing tasks.

What we have seen from the discussion of the two excerpts is that talk was deeply embedded in a complex interactional work between the co-present parties. This complex interactional work was the social organization through which sense-making was accomplished. Giving information was an activity that involved, among other things, finding the proper places where the information was to be found, orienting to the new configuration of relevancies in place, shifting the engagement from one task to another. Each operator made clear to his/her colleague the path, direction and issues at stake (what to say, who would say it, what was happening, who should do what) by means of various devices (the positioning of their bodies, pointing, the design of the talk addressed to his/her colleague, etc.). All this interactional work was deleted by the official audio recording of the events. Instead, the video recordings granted access to a whole interactional backstage (Goodwin, 1995) necessary for producing the official communication as it was. The backstage is an important place, not for ritual demands (as for Goffman), but for the structure itself of the service. At the call and dispatch centre, the booth was a place of intense cooperation and collaboration, through bodily and verbal means, explicit or tacit, between physically co-present persons, in order to provide a service, given the temporal constraints of the actual situation in which the operators concretely were. Official communications are the result of a process of social interaction between people who work together and share the same ecology, the same orientation and the same priorities, and who jointly ensure the alignment and concordance of that ecology, that orientation and those priorities.

Incoming phone calls and radio calls were not heard solely by the receiver but also by all those in the vicinity: everyone within earshot could listen to the communication without the use of any special devices. Incoming phone and radio calls enabled the operators present in the booth to overhear and monitor the ongoing activity, often while other activities were in progress. The operators were able to assess the importance of the incoming phone and radio calls and act accordingly. We have seen how the phone and radio calls created a sound environment that triggered simultaneous courses of action by those present and enabled their co-participation in joint work on a specific task.

References

Büscher, M. (2005). Social life under the microscope? *Sociological Research Online, 10*(1), 100–123.

Clawson, J. J., & Dernocoeur, K. B. (1988). *Principles of emergency medical dispatch.* Prentice Hall.

Dovigo, F., & Redaelli, I. (2007). *Ordinarie emergenze. Gruppi, tecnologie e storie del 118.* Guerini.

Dovigo, F., & Redaelli, I. (2010). Knowledge management in locating the patient in an emergency medical service in Italy. *Computer Supported Cooperative Work (CSCW), 19*(5), 457–481.

Falzon, P. A. (2009). Discourse segmentation and the management of multiple tasks in single episodes of air traffic controllerpilot spoken radio communication. *Discours 4.* http://journals.openedition.org/discours/7241

Fele, G. (2008). The collaborative production of responses and dispatching on the radio: Video analysis in a medical emergency call center. *Forum Qualitative Sozialforschung/Forum: Qualitative Social Research, 9*(3). https://doi.org/10.17169/fqs-9.3.1175

Fele, G. (2012). The use of video to document tacit participation in an emergency operations centre. *Qualitative Research, 12*(3), 280–303.

Gobo, G., Rozzi, S., Zanini, S., & Diotti, A. (2008). Routine dell'emergenza: il caso del 118. In S. Gherardi (Ed.), *Apprendimento tecnologico e tecnologie di apprendimento* (pp. 209–239). Il Mulino.

Goffman, E. (1979). Footing. *Semiotica, 25*(1–2), 1–29.

Goodwin, M. H. (1995). Assembling a response: Setting and collaboratively constructed work talk. In P. ten Have & G. Psathas (Eds.), *Situated order: Studies in the social organization of talk and embodied activities* (pp. 173–186). University Press of America.

Goodwin, C., & Goodwin, M. H. (1996). Formulating planes: Seeing as a situated activity. In Y. Engestrom & D. Middleton (Eds.), *Cognition and communication at work* (pp. 61–95). Cambridge University Press.

Heath, C., & Luff, P. (2006). Video analysis and organizational practice. In H. Knoblauch, B. Schnettler, J. Raab, & H. G. Soeffner (Eds.), *Video analysis: Methodology and methods* (pp. 35–49). Peter Lang.

Heath, C., Hindmarsh, J., & Luff, P. (2010). *Video in qualitative research. Analyzing social interaction in everyday life*. Sage.

Hedman, K. (2016). *Managing medical emergency calls* (Doctoral dissertation, Lund University Open Access).

Hénault-Tessier, M., & Dalle-Nazébi, S. (2012). Traiter les appels d'urgence. Fabriquer une information pour l'action. *Revue d'anthropologie des connaissances, 6*(6–1), 89–114.

Kevoe-Feldman, H. (2019). Inside the emergency service call-center: Reviewing thirty years of language and social interaction research. *Research on Language and Social Interaction, 52*(3), 227–240.

Kevoe-Feldman, H., & Pomerantz, A. (2018). Critical timing of actions for transferring 911 calls in a wireless call center. *Discourse Studies, 20*(4), 488–505.

Knoblauch, H. (2006). Videography. Focused ethnography and video analysis. In H. Knoblauch, B. Schnettler, J. Raab, & H. G. Soeffner (Eds.), *Video analysis: Methodology and methods* (pp. 69–83). Peter Lang.

Knoblauch, H., & Schnettler, B. (2012). Videography: Analysing video data as a 'focused' ethnographic and hermeneutical exercise. *Qualitative Research, 12*(3), 334–356.

Licoppe, C., & Relieu, M. (2005). Entre système et conversation. Une approche située de la compétence des téléopérateurs dans les services d'assistance technique. In E. Kessous & J.-L. Metzger (Eds.), *Le travail avec les technologies de l'information* (pp. 177–199). Hermès.

Luff, P., & Heath, C. (2002). Broadcast talk: Initiating calls through a computer-mediated technology. *Research on Language and Social Interaction, 35*(3), 337–366.

Luff, P., Hindmarsh, J., & Heath, C. (Eds.). (2000). *Workplace studies: Recovering work practice and informing system design*. Cambridge University Press.

Mellinger, W. M. (1992). Accomplishing fact in police "dispatch packages": An analysis for the situated construction of an organizational record. In G. Miller & J. A. Holstein (Eds.), *Perspectives on social problems* (Vol. 4, pp. 47–72). JAI Press.

Mellinger, W. M. (1994). Negotiated orders: The negotiation of directives in paramedic-nurse interaction. *Symbolic Interaction, 17*(2), 165–185.

Mondada, L. (2006). Video recording as the preservation of fundamental features for analysis. In H. Knoblauch, B. Schnettler, J. Raab, & H. G. Soeffner (Eds.), *Video analysis: Methodology and methods* (pp. 51–67). Peter Lang.

Mondada, L. (2008). Using video for a sequential and multimodal analysis of social interaction: Videotaping institutional telephone calls. *Forum Qualitative Sozialforschung/Forum: Qualitative Social Research, 9*(3). https://doi.org/10.17169/fqs-9.3.1161

Mondada, L. (2014). The local constitution of multimodal resources for social interaction. *Journal of Pragmatics, 65*, 137–156.

Mondada, L. (2018). Multiple temporalities of language and body in interaction: Challenges for transcribing multimodality. *Research on Language and Social Interaction, 51*(1), 85–106.

Mondada, L. (2022). The situated and methodic production of accountable action. The challenges of multimodality. In D. W. Maynard & J. Heritage (Eds.), *The ethnomethodology program. Legacies and prospects* (pp. 289–321). Oxford University Press.

Paoletti, I. (2009). Communication and diagnostic work in medical emergency calls in Italy. *Computer Supported Cooperative Work (CSCW), 18*(2), 229–250.

Rautiainen, I., Haddington, P., & Kamunen, A. (2022). Local participation framework as a resource among military observer trainees: Interactional episodes between repair initiation and repair solution in critical radio communication. *Journal of Pragmatics, 196*, 67–85.

Relieu, M., Licoppe, C., & Lan Hing Ting, K. (2010). Filmer le travail dans les centres d'appels: le cadrage vidéo et sonore comme mise à l'échelle de l'activité. In G. Valléry, M.-C. Le Port, & M. Zouinar (Eds.), *Ergonomie, conception de produits et services médiatisés* (pp. 37–55). Presses Universitaires de France.

Rollet, N. (2012). *Analyse conversationnelle des pratiques dans les appels au SAMU-Centre 115: Vers une approche praxéologique d'une forme située 'd'accord'.*. PhD thesis, Université de la Sorbonne nouvelle—Paris III.

Sanders, R. E. (2003). Conversational socializing on marine VHF radio: Adapting laughter and other practices to the technology in use. In P.J. Glenn, C.D. LeBaron & J. S. Mandelbaum (Eds.), *Studies in language and social interaction* (pp. 309–326). Lawrence Erlbaum Ass.

Simmons, J. L. (1974). *Efficient conversation: The talk between pilots and air traffic controllers.* Department of Sociology, University of Colorado. https://files.eric.ed.gov/fulltext/ED088296.pdf

Strevens, P. (1984). International maritime English (seaspeak). *Special Language-Fachsprache, 6*(1–2), 2–10.

Szymanski, M. H., Vinkhuyzen, E., Aoki, P. M., & Woodruff, A. (2006). Organizing a remote state of incipient talk: Push-to-talk mobile radio interaction. *Language in Society, 35*(3), 393–418.

Tjora, A. (2000). The technological mediation of the nursing-medical boundary. *Sociology of Health & Illness, 22*(6), 721–741.

Tjora, A. (2004). Maintaining redundancy in the coordination of medical emergencies. In *Proc. of the 2004 ACM Conf. on Computer Supported Cooperative Work*. ACM Press.

Tjora, A. (2009). *Calls for care. Coordination, competence, and computers in medical emergency call centres.* VDM Verlag.

Tuncer, S. (2016). The effects of video recording on office workers' conduct, and the validity of video data for the study of naturally-occurring interactions. *Forum Qualitative Sozialforschung/Forum: Qualitative Social Research, 17*(3), Art. 7. http://nbn-resolving.de/urn:nbn:de:0114-fqs160373

Whalen, J., & Zimmerman, D. H. (2005). Working a call: Multiparty management and interactional infrastructure in calls for help. In C. D. Baker, M. Emmison, & A. Firth (Eds.), *Calling for help. Language and social interaction in telephone helplines* (pp. 309–345). John Benjamins.

Wong, B. L. W., & Blandford, A. (2001). Situation awareness and its implications for human–systems interaction. In W. Smith, R. Thomas, et al. (Eds.), *Proc. of the Australian Conf. on computer-human interaction 2001* (pp. 181–186). Ergonomics Society of Australia.

Wong, B. L. W., & Blandford, A. (2002). Analysing ambulance dispatcher decision making: Trialing emergent themes analysis. *Proc. HF2002.* https://discovery.ucl.ac.uk/id/eprint/16628/1/16628.pdf

Appendix

Symbols Used for the Transcription

[	Left brackets indicate the point at which a current speaker's talk is overlapped by another's talk.
]	Right brackets indicate the point at which two overlapping utterances end.
=	Equals signs, one at the end of a line and one at the beginning, indicate no gap between the two lines.
(0.4)	Numbers in parentheses indicate elapsed time in silence in tenths of a second.
(.)	A dot in parentheses indicates a tiny gap, probably no more than one-tenth of a second.
______	Underscoring indicates some form of stress via pitch and/or amplitude.
::	Colons indicate prolongation of the immediately-prior sound. The length of the row of colons indicates the length of the prolongation.
WORD	Capitals, except at the beginnings of lines, indicate especially loud sounds relative to the surrounding talk.
.hhhh	A row of hs prefixed by a dot indicates an inbreath; without a dot, an outbreath. The length of the row of hs indicates the length of the in- or outbreath.

G. Fele, *Emergency Communication*,
https://doi.org/10.1007/978-3-031-26239-5

( )	Empty parentheses indicate the transcriber's inability to hear what was said.
(word)	Parenthesized words are possible hearings.
(( ))	Double parentheses contain author's descriptions rather than transcriptions.
-	A hyphen after a word or part of a word indicates a cut-off or self-interruption, often done with a glottal or a dental stop.
°	The degree sign indicates that the talk following it was markedly quiet or soft.
> <	"Greater than" and "less than" carrots? in this order indicate that the talk between them is rushed or compressed.
< >	"Less than" and "greater than" carrots? in this order indicate that the talk between them is markedly slow.
↓ or ↑	The up and down arrows mark sharp rises or falls in pitch or may mark a whole shift or resetting of the pitch.

References

Albert, S., Housley, W., & Stokoe, E. (2019). In case of emergency, order pizza. An urgent case of action formation and recognition. In *1st International Conference on Conversational User Interfaces (CUI 2019)*, August 22–23, 2019, Dublin, Ireland. ACM, New York. https://doi.org/10.1145/3342775.3342800

Antunes, G., & Scott, E. J. (1981). Calling the cops: Police telephone operators and citizen calls for service. *Journal of Criminal Justice, 9*, 165–179.

Arminen, I. (2005). *Institutional interaction: Studies of talk at work*. Ashgate.

Arminen, I. (2006). Social functions of location in mobile telephony. *Personal and Ubiquitous Computers, 10*, 319–323.

Arminen, I., & Leinonen, M. (2006). Mobile phone call openings: Tailoring answers to personalized summonses. *Discourse Studies, 8*(3), 339–368.

Baker, C., Emmison, M., & Firth, A. (Eds.). (2005). *Calling for help: Language and social interaction in telephone helplines*. John Benjamins.

Baraldi, C., & Gavioli, L. (2012). Introduction: Understanding coordination in interpreter-mediated interaction. In C. Baraldi & L. Gavioli (Eds.), *Coordinating participation in dialogue interpreting* (pp. 1–21). John Benjamins.

Bauer, A. M., & Alegría, M. (2010). Impact of patient language proficiency and interpreter service use on the quality of psychiatric care: A systematic review. *Psychiatric Services, 61*(8), 765–773.

Baumgarten, N., & House, J. (2010). I think and I don't know in English as lingua franca and native English discourse. *Journal of Pragmatics, 42*(5), 1184–1200.

G. Fele, *Emergency Communication*,
https://doi.org/10.1007/978-3-031-26239-5

Beach, W. A., & Metzger, T. R. (1997). Claiming insufficient knowledge. *Human Communication Research, 23*(4), 562–588.

Bercal, T. E. (1970). Calls for police assistance: Consumer demands for governmental service. *American Behavioral Scientist, 13*, 681–691.

Berdowski, J., Beekhuis, F., Zwinderman, A. H., Tijssen, J. G., & Koster, R. W. (2009). Importance of the first link: Description and recognition of an out-of-hospital cardiac arrest in an emergency call. *Circulation, 119*(15), 2096–2102.

Berger, I., Kitzinger, C., & Ellis, S. J. (2016). Using a category to accomplish resistance in the context of an emergency call: Michael Jackson's doctor. *Pragmatics, 26*(4), 563–582.

Bergmann, J. R. (1992). Alarmiertes Verstehen: Kommunikation in Feuerwehrnotrufen. In T. Jung & S. Müller-Doohm (Eds.), *"Wirklichkeit" im Deutungsprozeß. Verstehen und Methoden in den Kultur- und Sozialwissenschaften* (pp. 283–328). Suhrkamp.

Betz, E., & Deppermann, A. (2021). OKAY in responding and claiming understanding. In E. Betz, A. Deppermann, L. Mondada, & M.-L. Sorjonen (Eds.), *OKAY across languages: Toward a comparative approach to its use in talk-in-interaction* (pp. 55–92). John Benjamins.

Bloch, S., & Leydon, G. (2019). Conversation analysis and telephone helplines for health and illness: A narrative review. *Research on Language and Social Interaction, 52*(3), 193–211.

Bolaños-Carpio, A. (2020). When emergencies are not urgent: Requesting help in calls to the 9-1-1 Costa Rica. In C. Taleghani-Nikazm, E. Betz, & P. Golato (Eds.), *Mobilizing others: Grammar and lexis within larger activities* (pp. 229–252). John Benjamins Publishing Company.

Bolaños-Carpio, A. (2021). Place formulation in an emergency: The case of 911 calls in Costa Rica. *Language & Communication, 80*, 80–94.

Booker, M. J., Shaw, A. R., Purdy, S., & Barnes, R. (2018). 'Primary care sensitive' situations that result in an ambulance attendance: A conversation analytic study of UK emergency '999' call recordings. *BMJ Open, 8*(11), e023727.

Bradley, S. M., Fahrenbruch, C. E., Meischke, H., Allen, J., Bloomingdale, M., & Rea, T. D. (2011). Bystander CPR in out-of-hospital cardiac arrest: The role of limited English proficiency. *Resuscitation, 82*(6), 680–684.

Broadhead, R. S. (1986). Directing intervention from afar: The telephone dynamics of managing acute poisoning. *Journal of Health and Social Behavior, 27*, 303–319.

Burke, P. (2006). The hybridization of languages in early modern Europe. *European Review, 14*(1), 105–110.

Büscher, M. (2005a). Embodied conduct and movement in emergency teamwork. In L. Mondada (Ed.), *Gestures and the organisation of social interaction: Ethnomethodological and conversational perspectives.* Conference Proceedings. Lyon-France June 15–18. https://eprints.lancs.ac.uk/id/eprint/62088/1/Buscher_revised2706.pdf

Büscher, M. (2005b). Social life under the microscope? *Sociological Research Online, 10*(1), 100–123.

Carroll, L. N., Calhoun, R. E., Subido, C. C., Painter, I. S., & Meischke, H. W. (2013). Serving limited English proficient callers: A survey of 9-1-1 police telecommunicators. *Prehospital and Disaster Medicine, 28*(3), 286–291.

Chapman, S., & Schofield, W. N. (1998). Lifesavers and samaritans: Emergency use of cellular (mobile) phones in Australia. *Accident Analysis & Prevention, 30*(6), 815–819.

Clawson, J. J., & Dernocoeur, K. B. (1988). *Principles of emergency medical dispatch*. Prentice Hall.

Clayman, S. E., & Heritage, J. (2014). Benefactor and beneficiaries. In P. Drew & E. Couper-Kuhlen (Eds.), *Requesting in social interaction* (pp. 55–86). John Benjamins.

Clayman, S. E., Heritage, J., & Maynard, D. W. (2022). The ethnomethodological lineage of conversation analysis. In D. W. Maynard & J. Heritage (Eds.), *The ethnomethodology program: Legacies and prospects* (pp. 252–286). Oxford University Press.

Couper-Kuhlen, E. (2014). What does grammar tell us about action? *Pragmatics, 24*(3), 623–647.

Crabtree, A., O'Neill, J., Tolmie, P., Castellani, S., Colombino, T., & Grasso, A. (2006). The practical indispensability of articulation work to immediate and remote help-giving. In *CSCW '06: Proceedings of the 2006 20th anniversary conference on Computer supported cooperative work* November, 219–228. https://doi.org/10.1145/1180875.1180910

Craven, A., & Potter, J. (2010). Directives: Entitlement and contingency in action. *Discourse Studies, 12*(4), 419–442.

Cromdal, J. (2012). Conversation analysis and emergency calls. In C. Chapelle (Ed.), *The encyclopaedia of applied linguistics*. Wiley-Blackwell.

Cromdal, J., Osvaldsson, K., & Persson-Thunqvist, D. (2008). Context that matters: Producing "thick-enough descriptions" in initial emergency reports. *Journal of Pragmatics, 40*(5), 927–959.

Cromdal, J., Landqvist, H., Persson-Thunqvist, D., & Osvaldsson, K. (2012a). Finding out what's happened: Two procedures for opening emergency calls. *Discourse Studies, 14*(4), 371–397.

Cromdal, J., Persson-Thunqvist, D., & Osvaldsson, K. (2012b). "SOS 112 what has occurred?" Managing openings in children's emergency calls. *Discourse, Context & Media, 1*(4), 183–202.

Curl, T. S., & Drew, P. (2008). Contingency and action: A comparison of two forms of requesting. *Research on Language and Social Interaction, 41*(2), 129–153.

Danby, S., Baker, C., & Emmison, M. (2005). Four observations on openings in calls to kids help line. In C. D. Baker, M. Emmison, & A. Firth (Eds.), *Calling for help. Language and social interaction in telephone helplines* (pp. 133–151). Benjamins.

Danby, S., Butler, C. W., & Emmison, M. (2009). When "listeners can't talk": Comparing active listening in opening sequences of telephone and online counselling. *Australian Journal of Communication, 36*(3), 91–114.

De Stefani, E. (2018). Formulating direction: Navigational instructions in driving lessons. *International Journal of Applied Linguistics, 28*(2), 283–303.

Deppermann, A. (2011). The study of formulations as key to an interactional semantics. *Human Studies, 34*(2), 115–128.

Deppermann, A., & Gubina, A. (2021). Positionally-sensitive action-ascription: Uses of Kannst du X? 'Can you X?' in their sequential and multimodal context. *Interactional Linguistics, 1*(2), 183–215.

Deppermann, A., & Haugh, M. (Eds.). (2022). *Action ascription in interaction.* Cambridge University Press.

Diani, G. (2004). The discourse functions of "I don't know" in English conversation. In K. Aijmer & A. Strenström (Eds.), *Discourse patterns in spoken and written corpora* (pp. 157–171). John Benjamins.

Dovigo, F., & Redaelli, I. (2007). *Ordinarie emergenze. Gruppi, tecnologie e storie del 118.* Guerini.

Dovigo, F., & Redaelli, I. (2010). Knowledge management in locating the patient in an emergency medical service in Italy. *Computer Supported Cooperative Work (CSCW), 19*(5), 457–481.

Drew, P. (1992). Contested evidence in courtroom cross-examination: The case of a trial for rape. In P. Drew & J. Heritage (Eds.), *Talk at work* (pp. 470–520). Cambridge University Press.

Drew, P. (1998). Out of hours calls to the doctor: Misalignment between callers and doctor during diagnostic questioning. In S. Cmejrkova, J. Hoffmannová, O. Müllerová, & J. Světlá (Eds.), *Dialoganalyse VI/2: Referate der 6. Arbeitstagung, Prag 1996* (pp. 65–78). Max Niemeyer Verlag.

Drew, P. (2003a). Comparative analysis of talk-in-interaction in different institutional settings: A sketch. In P. Glenn, C. LeBaron, & J. Mandelbaum (Eds.), *Studies in language and social interaction: In honor of Robert Hopper* (pp. 293–308). Lawrence Erlbaum.

Drew, P. (2003b). Precision and exaggeration in interaction. *American Sociological Review, 68*(6), 917–938.

Drew, P. (2006). Mis-alignments in 'after-hours' calls to a British GP's practice: A study in telephone medicine. In J. Heritage & D. W. Maynard (Eds.), *Communication in medical care: Interaction between primary care physicians and patients* (pp. 416–444). Cambridge University Press.

Drew, P. (2022). The micro-politics of social actions. In A. Deppermann & M. Haugh (Eds.), *Action ascription in social interaction* (pp. 57–82). Cambridge University Press.

Drew, P., & Couper-Kuhlen, E. (2014). Requesting—From speech act to recruitment. In P. Drew & E. Couper-Kuhlen (Eds.), *Requesting in social interaction* (pp. 1–34). John Benjamins.

Drew, P., & Heritage, J. (1992). Talk at work: An introduction. In P. Drew & J. Heritage (Eds.), *Talk at work: Interaction in institutional settings* (pp. 3–65). Cambridge University Press.

Drew, P., & Walker, T. (2010). Citizen's emergency calls to police: Requesting assistance in calls to the police. In M. Coulthard & A. Johnson (Eds.), *Handbook of forensic linguistic* (pp. 95–110). Routledge.

Eglin, P., & Wideman, D. (1986). Inequality in professional service encounters: Verbal strategies of control versus task performance in calls to the police. *Zeitschrift fur Soziologie, 15*(5), 341–362.

Elliot, H. C. (1974). Similarities and differences between science and common science. In R. Turner (Ed.), *Ethnomethodology. Selected readings* (pp. 21–26). Penguin.

Emerson, R. M. (1981). On last resorts. *The American Journal of Sociology, 87*(1), 1–22.

Emmison, M., & Danby, S. (2007). "Who's the friend in the background?": Interactional strategies in determining authenticity in calls to a national children's helpline. *Australian Review of Applied Linguistics, 30*(3), 31–31.

Eriksson, M. (2010). Conceptions of emergency calls: Emergency communication in an age of mobile communication and prevalence of anxiety. *Journal of Contingencies and Crisis Management, 18*(3), 165–174.

Falzon, P. A. (2009). Discourse segmentation and the management of multiple tasks in single episodes of air traffic controller-pilot spoken radio communication. *Discours 4.* http://journals.openedition.org/discours/7241

Fele, G. (2006). La communication dans l'urgence. Les appels au secours téléphoniques. *Revue française de linguistique appliquée, 11*(2), 33–51.

Fele, G. (2007). La rinuncia all'agency: forme di cooperazione e di interazione sociale tra gli operatori dell'emergenza. In A. Donzelli & A. Fasulo (Eds.), *Agency e linguaggio: etnoteorie della soggettività e della responsabilità nell'azione sociale* (pp. 173–193). Meltemi.

Fele, G. (2008). The collaborative production of responses and dispatching on the radio: Video analysis in a medical emergency call center. *Forum Qualitative Sozialforschung/Forum: Qualitative Social Research, 9*(3). https://doi.org/10.17169/fqs-9.3.1175

Fele, G. (2009). Glosse e formulazioni. In L. Mariottini, M. E. Sciubba, & M. Fatigante (Eds.), *Lingua e società. Scritti in onore di Franca Orletti per il suo sessantesimo compleanno* (pp. 49–59). Franco Angeli.

Fele, G. (2012). The use of video to document tacit participation in an emergency operations centre. *Qualitative Research, 12*(3), 280–303.

Fele, G. (2014a). Requesting help with null or limited knowledge. In A. Zuczkowski, R. Bongelli, I. Riccioni, & C. Canestrari (Eds.), *Communicating certainty and uncertainty in medical, supportive and scientific contexts* (pp. 139–156). John Benjamins.

Fele, G. (2014b). Stati interni e cognizione: che cosa facciamo quando parliamo con qualcuno. In L. Muzzetto (Ed.), *Wittgenstein e il pensiero sociologico* (pp. 189–212). Pisa.

Fele, G. (2016). Overcoming language barriers in emergency telephone calls. In A. F. Plastina (Ed.), *Challenging language barriers in the public service. An interdisciplinary perspective* (pp. 15–38). Aracne editrice.

Flores, G., Laws, M. B., Mayo, S. J., Zuckerman, B., Abreu, M., Medina, L., & Hardt, E. J. (2003). Errors in medical interpretation and their potential clinical consequences in paediatric encounters. *Pediatrics, 111*(1), 6–14.

Flores, G., Abreu, M., Barone, C. P., Bachur, R., & Lin, H. (2012). Errors of medical interpretation and their potential clinical consequences: A comparison of professional versus ad hoc versus no interpreters. *Annals of Emergency Medicine, 60*(5), 545–553.

Fox, B. A., & Heinemann, T. (2021). Are they requests? An exploration of declaratives of trouble in service encounters. *Research on Language and Social Interaction, 54*(1), 20–38.

Francis, D., & Hester, S. (2004). *An invitation to ethnomethodology: Language, society and social interaction*. Sage.

Frankel, R. M. (1989). "I wz wondering—uhm could Raid uhm effect the brain permanently d'y know?": Some observations on the intersection of speaking and writing in calls to a poison control center. *Western Journal of Speech Communication, 53*, 195–226.

Fussell, P. (2002). *Uniforms. Why we are what we wear*. Houghton Mifflin.

Garcia, A. C. (2013a). Routine service calls: Emergency calls to the police. In A. C. Garcia (Ed.), *An introduction to interaction: Understanding talk in formal and informal settings* (pp. 154–165). Bloomsbury.

Garcia, A. C. (2013b). Problematic emergency service calls. In A. C. Garcia (Ed.), *An introduction to interaction. Understanding talk in formal and informal settings* (pp. 166–182). Bloomsbury.

Garcia, A. C. (2015). 'Something really weird has happened': Losing the 'big picture' in emergency service calls. *Journal of Pragmatics, 84*, 102–120.

Garcia, A. C. (2017). What went right: Interactional strategies for managing crisis negotiations during an emergency service call. *The Sociological Quarterly, 58*(3), 495–518.

Garcia, A. C. (2022a). Interactional challenges for non-native speakers of English in emergency telephone calls. *Journal of Pragmatics, 193*, 222–234.

Garcia, A. C. (2022b). A preliminary investigation of the use of racial/ethnic categories in emergency telephone calls in the United States. *Journal of Applied Communication Research, 50*(4), 345–362.

Garcia, A. C., & Parmer, P. A. (1999). Misplaced mistrust: The collaborative construction of doubt in 911 emergency calls. *Symbolic Interaction, 22*(4), 297–324.

Garfinkel, H. (1967). *Studies in ethnomethodology*. Prentice-Hall.

Garfinkel, H. (2022). *Harold Garfinkel: Studies of work in the sciences* (M. Lynch, Ed.). Routledge.

Garfinkel, H., & Sacks, H. (1970). On formal structures of practical actions. In C. Mckinney & E. A. Tiryakian (Eds.), *Theoretical sociology* (pp. 338–366). Appleton Crofts.

Gavioli, L. (2012). Minimal responses in interpreter-mediated medical talk. In C. Baraldi & L. Gavioli (Eds.), *Coordinating participation in dialogue interpreting* (pp. 201–249). John Benjamins Publishing.

Gavioli, L., & Baraldi, C. (2011). Interpreter-mediated interaction in healthcare and legal settings: Talk organization, context and the achievement of intercultural communication. *Interpreting, 13*(2), 205–233.

Gerwing, J. (2015). Emergency telephone discourse. In K. Tracy, C. Ilie, & T. Sandel (Eds.), *The international encyclopedia of language and social interaction*. Wiley-Blackwell.

Gerwing, J., & Indseth, T. (2010). Communication with non-native callers in medical emergency calls. https://www.fhi.no/globalassets/dokumenterfiler/rapporter/2010/communication-with-non-native-callers-in-medical-emergency-calls.pdf

Gerwing, J., & Indseth, T. (2016). Enhancing caller comprehensibility in emergency calls with a language barrier: Operators in the role of addressee. *International Journal of Listening, 30*(3), 163–179.

Gilsinan, J. F. (1989). They is clowning tough: 911 and the social construction of reality. *Criminology, 27*(2), 329–344.

Gobo, G., Rozzi, S., Zanini, S., & Diotti, A. (2008). Routine dell'emergenza: il caso del 118. In S. Gherardi (Ed.), *Apprendimento tecnologico e tecnologie di apprendimento* (pp. 209–239). Il Mulino.

Goffman, E. (1979). Footing. *Semiotica, 25*(1–2), 1–29.

Goffman, E. (1981). *Forms of talk*. University of Pennsylvania Press.

Goffman, E. (1983). The interaction order. *American Sociological Review, 48*, 1–17.

González-Martínez, E. (2008). Des réponses "je ne sais pas" lors d'une enquête sociale. *Bulletin suisse de linguistique appliquée, 88*, 19–41.

González-Martínez, E. (2017). Ouverture d'appels téléphoniques infirmière-transporteur à l'hôpital. *Revue française de linguistique appliquée, 22*(2), 165–183.

González-Martínez, E., & Drew, P. (2021). Informings as recruitment in nurses' intrahospital telephone calls. *Journal of Pragmatics, 186*, 48–59.

Goodwin, M. H. (1995). Assembling a response: Setting and collaboratively constructed work talk. In P. ten Have & G. Psathas (Eds.), *Situated order: Studies in the social organization of talk and embodied activities* (pp. 173–186). University Press of America.

Goodwin, C. (1996). Transparent vision. In E. A. Schegloff, E. Ochs, & S. A. Thompson (Eds.), *Interaction and grammar* (pp. 370–404). Cambridge University Press.

Goodwin, C., & Goodwin, M. H. (1996). Formulating planes: Seeing as a situated activity. In Y. Engestrom & D. Middleton (Eds.), *Cognition and communication at work* (pp. 61–95). Cambridge University Press.

Grant, L. E. (2010). A corpus comparison of the use of "I don't know" by British and New Zealand speakers. *Journal of Pragmatics, 42*(8), 2282–2296.

Greco, L. (2004). Descriptions, catégories et collections de catégories. Le rôle de l'urgence dans le pratiques de catégorisation de la douleur dans les appels au 115. *Rivista di psicolinguistica applicate, 4*(2–3), 1–15.

Grice, P. (1975). Logic and conversation. In P. Cole & J. Morgan (Eds.), *Syntax and semantics. Vol. 3: Speech acts* (pp. 41–58). Academic Press.

Haddington, P., & Keisanen, T. (2009). Location, mobility and the body as resources in selecting a route. *Pragmatics, 41*(10), 1938–1961.

Haffner, L. (1992). Translation is not enough. Interpreting in a medical setting. *Western Journal of Medicine, 157*(3), 255.

Hayashi, R. (2019). Categorization for occasioned semantics: Reanalysis of a Japanese Yamagata 119 emergency call. *Discourse Studies, 21*(5), 495–521.

Hayashi, M., Raymond, G., & Sidnell, J. (2013). Conversational repair and human understanding: An introduction. In M. Hayashi, G. Raymond, & J. Sidnell (Eds.), *Conversational repair and human understanding* (pp. 1–30). Cambridge University Press.

Heath, C., & Luff, P. (1992). Collaboration and control. Crisis management and multimedia technology in London Underground Line Control Rooms. *Computer Supported Cooperative Work (CSCW), 1*(1), 69–94.

Heath, C., & Luff, P. (1996). Convergent activities: Line control and passenger information on the London underground. In Y. Engestrom & D. Middleton (Eds.), *Cognition and communication at work* (pp. 96–129). Cambridge University Press.

Heath, C., & Luff, P. (2000). *Technology in action.* Cambridge University Press.

Heath, C., & Luff, P. (2006). Video analysis and organizational practice. In H. Knoblauch, B. Schnettler, J. Raab, & H. G. Soeffner (Eds.), *Video analysis: Methodology and methods* (pp. 35–49). Peter Lang.

Heath, C., Knoblauch, H., & Luff, P. (2000). Technology and social interaction: The emergence of Workplace Studies. *British Journal of Sociology, 51*(2), 299–320.

Heath, C., Hindmarsh, J., & Luff, P. (2010). *Video in qualitative research. Analyzing social interaction in everyday life.* Sage.

Hedman, K. (2016). *Managing medical emergency calls* (Doctoral dissertation, Lund University Open Access).

Hénault-Tessier, M., & Dalle-Nazébi, S. (2012). Traiter les appels d'urgence. Fabriquer une information pour l'action. *Revue d'anthropologie des connaissances, 6*(6–1), 89–114.

Hepburn, A. (2005). "You're not takin' me seriously": Ethics and asymmetry in calls to a child protection helpline. *Journal of Constructivist Psychology, 18*, 253–274.

Hepburn, A., & Bolden, G. B. (2013). The conversation analytic approach to transcription. In J. Sidnell & T. Stivers (Eds.), *The handbook of conversation analysis* (pp. 57–76). Wiley-Blackwell Publishing.

Hepburn, A., Wilkinson, S., & Butler, C. W. (2014). Intervening with conversation analysis in telephone helpline services: Strategies to improve effectiveness. *Research on Language and Social Interaction, 47*(3), 239–254.

Heritage, J. (1984). Conversation analysis. In J. Heritage (Ed.), *Garfinkel and ethnomethodology* (pp. 233–244). Polity Press.

Heritage, J. (2007). Intersubjectivity and progressivity in person (and place) reference. In T. Stivers & N. J. Enfield (Eds.), *Person reference in interaction: Linguistic, cultural, and social perspectives* (pp. 255–280). Cambridge University Press.

Heritage, J. (2013). Epistemics in conversation. In J. Sidnell & T. Stivers (Eds.), *Handbook of conversation analysis* (pp. 659–673). Wiley-Blackwell.

Heritage, J., & Clayman, S. E. (2010). Calls for emergency service. In J. Heritage & S. Clayman (Eds.), *Talk in action: Interactions, identities, and institutions* (pp. 53–100). Wiley-Blackwell.

Heritage, J., & Raymond, G. (2005). The terms of agreement: Indexing epistemic authority and subordination in talk-in-interaction. *Social Psychology Quarterly, 68*(1), 15–38.

Heritage, J., & Watson, D. (1979). Formulations as conversational objects. In G. Psathas (Ed.), *Everyday language: Studies in ethnomethodology* (pp. 123–162). Irvington.

Heritage, J., & Watson, D. (1980). Aspects of the properties of formulations in natural conversations: Some instances analysed. *Semiotica, 30*(3–4), 245–262.

Hindmarsh, J., & Heath, C. (2007). Video-based studies of work practice. *Sociology Compass, 1*(1), 156–173.

Holt, E. (2017). Indirect reported speech in storytelling: Its position, design, and uses. *Research on Language and Social Interaction, 50*(2), 171–187.

Houtkoop, H., Jansen, F., & Walstock, A. (2005). Collaborative problem description in help desk calls. In C. Baker, M. Emmison, & A. Firth (Eds.), *Calling for help: Language and social interaction in telephone helplines* (pp. 63–90). John Benjamins.

Hughes, E. C. (1971). *The sociological eye*. Aldine Atherton.

Hughes, D. (1980). The ambulance journey as an information generating process. *Sociology of Health and Illness, 2*(2), 115–132.

Hutchby, I. (2002). Resisting the incitement to talk in child counselling: Aspects of the utterance 'I don't know'. *Discourse Studies, 4*(2), 147–168.

Ikeya, N. (2003). Practical management of mobility: The case of the emergency medical system. *Environment and Planning A, 35*(9), 1547–1564.

Imbens-Bailey, A., & McCabe, A. (2000). The discourse of distress: A narrative analysis of emergency calls to 911. *Language and Communication, 20*, 275–296.

Iversen, C. (2021). Making sense of experiences in suicide helpline calls: Offering empathy without endorsing suicidal ideation. *Sociology of Health & Illness, 43*(9), 2066–2084.

Jacobs, E., Chen, A. H., Karliner, L. S., Agger-Gupta, N. I. E. L. S., & Mutha, S. (2006). The need for more research on language barriers in health care: A proposed research agenda. *The Milbank Quarterly, 84*(1), 111–133.

Jefferson, G. (1989). Preliminary notes on a possible metric which provides for a "standard maximum" silence of approximately one second in conversation. In D. Roger & P. Bull (Eds.), *Conversation: An interdisciplinary perspective* (pp. 166–196). Multilingual Matters.

Jefferson, G., & Lee, J. R. E. (1981). The rejection of advice: Managing the problematic convergence of a 'troubles-telling' and a 'service encounter'. *Journal of Pragmatics, 5*(5), 399–422.

Kale, E., & Syed, H. R. (2010). Language barriers and the use of interpreters in the public health services. A questionnaire-based survey. *Patient Education and Counseling, 81*(2), 187–191.

Kameo, N., & Whalen, J. (2015). Organizing documents: Standard forms, person production and organizational action. *Qualitative Sociology, 38*(2), 205–229.

Kärkkäinen, E. (2003). *Epistemic stance in English conversation: A description of its interactional functions, with a focus on 'I think'*. John Benjamins.

Kärkkäinen, E. (2006). Stance taking in conversation: From subjectivity to intersubjectivity. *Text and Talk, 26*(6), 699–731.

Karliner, L. S., Jacobs, E. A., Chen, A. H., & Mutha, S. (2007). Do professional interpreters improve clinical care for patients with limited English proficiency? A systematic review of the literature. *Health Services Research, 42*(2), 727–754.

Kazemi, A. (2020). Fine-tuning locational formulations in mobile phone calls. *Discourse Studies, 22*(5), 553–570.

Keevallik, L. (2011). The terms of not knowing and social affiliation. In T. Stivers, L. Mondada, & J. Steensig (Eds.), *The morality of knowledge in conversation* (pp. 184–206). Cambridge University Press.

Kent, A., & Antaki, C. (2020). Police call-takers' first substantive question projects the outcome of the call. *Applied Linguistics, 41*(5), 640–661.

Kevoe-Feldman, H. (2016). "Why are you concerned?" A consideration of turn distance and the organization of the interrogative series in "wellness check" calls to a university police department. *Discourse Processes, 53*(7), 556–580.

Kevoe-Feldman, H. (2019). Inside the emergency service call-center: Reviewing thirty years of language and social interaction research. *Research on Language and Social Interaction, 52*(3), 227–240.

Kevoe-Feldman, H., & Iversen, C. (2022). Approaching institutional boundaries: Comparative conversation analysis of practices for assisting suicidal callers in emergency and suicide helpline calls. *Journal of Pragmatics, 191*, 83–97.

Kevoe-Feldman, H., & Pomerantz, A. (2018). Critical timing of actions for transferring 911 calls in a wireless call center. *Discourse Studies, 20*(4), 488–505.

Kevoe-Feldman, H., & Sutherland, C. B. (2018). The "four-second rule" for identifying the active silent 911 caller. *Annals of Emergency Dispatch & Response, 6*(1), 5–9.

Kitzinger, C. (2011). Working with childbirth helplines: The contributions and limitations of conversation analysis. In C. Antaki (Ed.), *Applied conversation analysis: Intervention and change in institutional talk* (pp. 98–118). Palgrave Macmillan.

Kitzinger, C., Lerner, G. H., Zinken, J., Wilkinson, S., Kevoe-Feldman, H., & Ellis, S. (2013). Reformulating place. *Journal of Pragmatics, 55*, 43–50.

Knoblauch, H. (2006). Videography. Focused ethnography and video analysis. In H. Knoblauch, B. Schnettler, J. Raab, & H. G. Soeffner (Eds.), *Video analysis: Methodology and methods* (pp. 69–83). Peter Lang.

Knoblauch, H., & Schnettler, B. (2012). Videography: Analysing video data as a 'focused' ethnographic and hermeneutical exercise. *Qualitative Research, 12*(3), 334–356.

Koole, T., & van Burgsteden, L. (2022). Actions and identities in emergency calls: The case of thanking. In A. Deppermann & M. Haugh (Eds.), *Action ascription in interaction* (pp. 256–276). Cambridge University Press.

Koole, T., & Verberg, N. (2017). Aligning caller and call-taker: The opening phrase of Dutch emergency calls. *Pragmatics and Society, 8*(1), 129–153.

Labov, W., & Fanshel, D. (1977). *Therapeutic discourse: Psychotherapy as conversation*. Academic Press.

Lan Hing Ting, K. (2009). Ethnographier le bruit en centre d'appels. Une analyse située de l'activité des téléopérateurs. *Activités, 6*(6–2). http://journals.openedition.org/activites/2272. https://doi.org/10.4000/activites.2272

Landgren, J. (2005). Supporting fire crew sensemaking enroute to incidents. *International Journal of Emergency Management, 2*(3), 176–188.

Landgren, J., & Bergstrand, F. (2010). Mobile live video in emergency response: Its use and consequences. *Bulletin of the American Society for Information Science and Technology, 36*(5), 27–29.

Landgren, J., & Nulden, U. (2007). A study of emergency response work: Patterns of mobile phone interaction. In *Proceedings of the SIGCHI conference on Human factors in computing systems*, April, 1323–1332.

Larsen, T. (2013). Dispatching emergency assistance: Callers' claims of entitlement and call takers' decisions. *Research on Language and Social Interaction, 46*(3), 205–230.

Laurier, E. (2001). Why people say where they are during mobile phone calls. *Environment and Planning D: Society and Space, 19*(4), 485–504.

Lee, S. H. (2011a). Managing nongranting of customers' requests in commercial service encounters. *Research on Language and Social Interaction, 44*(2), 109–134.

Lee, S. H. (2011b). Responding at a higher level: Activity progressivity in calls for service. *Journal of Pragmatics, 43*(3), 904–917.

Leppänen, V. (2010). Power in telephone advice nursing. *Nursing Inquiry, 17*(1), 15–26.

Lerner, G. H., & Kitzinger, C. (2007). Extraction and aggregation in the repair of individual and collective self-reference. *Discourse Studies, 9*(4), 526–557.

Lerner, G. H., Bolden, G. B., Hepburn, A., & Mandelbaum, J. (2012). Granularity recalibration repairs: Refining formulations for the task at hand. *Research on Language and Social Interaction, 45*(2), 191–212.

Levinson, S. C. (1992). Activity types and language. In P. Drew & J. Heritage (Eds.), *Talk at work: Interaction in institutional settings* (pp. 66–100). Cambridge University Press.

Levinson, S. C. (1998). Minimization and conversational inference. In A. Kasher (Ed.), *Pragmatics: Vol. 4 Presupposition, implicature and indirect speech acts* (pp. 545–612). Routledge.

Leydon, G. M., Ekberg, K., & Drew, P. (2013). "How can I help?" Nurse call openings on a cancer helpline and implications for call progressivity. *Patient Education and Counseling, 92*(1), 23–30.

Liberman, K. (2012). The intelligibility of directions: The Psathas corpus. In H. Nasu & F. Chaput Waksler (Eds.), *Interaction and everyday life: Phenomenological and ethnomethodological essays in honor of George Psathas* (pp. 251–260). Lexington Books.

Liberman, K. (2013). Following sketched maps. In K. Liberman (Ed.), *More studies in ethnomethodology* (pp. 45–82). SUNY Press.

Licoppe, C., & Relieu, M. (2005). Entre système et conversation. Une approche située de la compétence des téléopérateurs dans les services d'assistance technique. In E. Kessous & J.-L. Metzger (Eds.), *Le travail avec les technologies de l'information* (pp. 177–199). Hermès.

Ludwig, T., Reuter, C., & Pipek, V. (2013). What you see is what I need: Mobile reporting practices in emergencies. In *ECSCW 2013: Proceedings of the 13th European Conference on Computer Supported Cooperative Work, 21–25 September 2013, Paphos, Cyprus* (pp. 181–206). Springer.

Luff, P., & Heath, C. (2002). Broadcast talk: Initiating calls through a computer-mediated technology. *Research on Language and Social Interaction, 35*(3), 337–366.

Luff, P., Hindmarsh, J., & Heath, C. (Eds.). (2000). *Workplace studies: Recovering work practice and informing system design*. Cambridge University Press.

Lynch, M. (2000). The ethnomethodological foundations of conversation analysis. *Text, 20*(4), 517–532.

Manning, P. F. (1988). *Symbolic communication. Signifying calls and the police response*. MIT Press.

Mannon, J. M. (1981). *Emergency encounters. A study of an ambulance service*. Kennikat Press.

Marquez Reiter, R. (2006). Interactional closeness in service calls to a Montevidean carer service company. *Research on Language and Social Interaction, 39*(1), 7–39.

Martin, D., O'Neill, J., Randall, D., & Rouncefield, M. (2007). How can I help you? Call centres, classification work and coordination. *Computer Supported Cooperative Work (CSCW), 16*(3), 231–264.

Mauss, M. (1921). L'expression obligatoire des sentiments (rituels oraux funéraires australiens). *Journal de psychologie, 18*, 425–434.

Maynard, D. W. (2013). Everyone and No one to turn to: Intellectual roots and contexts for conversation analysis. In J. Sidnell & T. Stivers (Eds.), *The handbook of conversation analysis* (pp. 11–31). Willey-Blackwell Publishing.

McCarthy, J. C., Wright, P. C., Healey, P., Dearden, A., & Harrison, M. D. (1997). Locating the scene: The particular and the general in contexts for ambulance control. In *Proceedings of the international ACM SIGGROUP conference on supporting group work: The integration challenge* (pp. 101–110). Phoenix, Arizona, United States.

McHoul, A. W., & Watson, D. R. (1984). Two axes for the analysis of 'commonsense' and 'formal' geographical knowledge in classroom talk. *British Journal of Sociology of Education, 5*(3), 281–302.

Meehan, A. J. (1989). Assessing the "police-worthiness" of citizen complaints to the police: Accountability and the negotiation of "facts". In D. T. Helm, W. T. Anderson, A. J. Meehan, & A. Rawls (Eds.), *The interactional order: New directions in the study of social order* (pp. 116–140). Irvington Publishers, Inc.

Meischke, H., Chavez, D., Bradley, S., Rea, T., & Eisenberg, M. (2010). Emergency communications with limited-English-proficiency populations. *Prehospital Emergency Care, 14*(2), 265–271.

Meischke, H. W., Calhoun, R. E., Yip, M. P., Tu, S. P., & Painter, I. S. (2013). The effect of language barriers on dispatching EMS response. *Prehospital Emergency Care, 17*(4), 475–480.

Meischke, H., Ike, B., Painter, I., Chavez, D., Yip, M. P., Bradley, S. M., & Tu, S.-P. (2015). Delivering 9-1-1 CPR instructions to limited English proficient callers: A simulation experiment. *Journal of Immigrant and Minority Health, 17*, 1049–1054.

Mellinger, W. M. (1992a). Talk-as-work: The case of paramedic calls for emergency field orders. *Current Research on Occupations and Professions, 7*, 79–109.

Mellinger, W. M. (1992b). Accomplishing fact in police "dispatch packages": An analysis for the situated construction of an organizational record. In G. Miller & J. A. Holstein (Eds.), *Perspectives on social problems* (Vol. 4, pp. 47–72). JAI Press.

Mellinger, W. M. (1994). Negotiated orders: The negotiation of directives in paramedic-nurse interaction. *Symbolic Interaction, 17*(2), 165–185.

Merritt, M. (1980). On the use of OK in service encounters. In E. W. Shuy & A. Shunkal (Eds.), *Language use and the uses of language* (pp. 162–172). Georgetown University Press.

Metz, D. L. (1981). *Running hot. Structure and stress in ambulance work.* ABT Books.

Mondada, L. (2006). Video recording as the preservation of fundamental features for analysis. In H. Knoblauch, B. Schnettler, J. Raab, & H. G. Soeffner (Eds.), *Video analysis: Methodology and methods* (pp. 51–67). Peter Lang.

Mondada, L. (2008). Using video for a sequential and multimodal analysis of social interaction: Videotaping institutional telephone calls. *Forum Qualitative Sozialforschung/Forum: Qualitative Social Research, 9*(3). https://doi.org/10.17169/fqs-9.3.1161

Mondada, L. (2010). Reassembling fragmented geographies. In M. Büscher, J. Urry, & K. Witchger (Eds.), *Mobile methods* (pp. 138–163). New York.

Mondada, L. (2011a). Géographies mobiles et divergentes. L'établissement interactionnel des lieux d'intervention dans des appels au secours. *Revue d'anthropologie des connaissances, 5*(2), 390–436.

Mondada, L. (2011b). The management of knowledge discrepancies and of epistemic changes in institutional interactions. In T. Stivers, L. Mondada, & J. Steensig (Eds.), *The morality of knowledge in conversation* (pp. 27–57). Cambridge University Press.

Mondada, L. (2014). The local constitution of multimodal resources for social interaction. *Journal of Pragmatics, 65*, 137–156.

Mondada, L. (2018). Multiple temporalities of language and body in interaction: Challenges for transcribing multimodality. *Research on Language and Social Interaction, 51*(1), 85–106.

Mondada, L. (2022). The situated and methodic production of accountable action. The challenges of multimodality. In D. W. Maynard & J. Heritage (Eds.), *The ethnomethodology program. Legacies and prospects* (pp. 289–321). Oxford University Press.

Mondada, L., & Sorjonen, M.-L. (2021). OKAY in closings and transitions. In E. Betz, A. Deppermann, L. Mondada, & M.-L. Sorjonen (Eds.), *OKAY across languages: Toward a comparative approach to its use in talk-in-interaction* (pp. 94–127). John Benjamins.

Monzoni, C. M. (2009a). Direct complaints in (Italian) calls to the ambulance: The use of negatively framed questions. *Journal of Pragmatics, 41*(12), 2465–2478.

Monzoni, C. M. (2009b). Preference organization and complaining in (Italian) 118 emergency calls to the ambulance. *Dialogue Analysis, XI*, 249–261.

Monzoni, C., & Zorzi, D. (2003). Le telefonate d'emergenza: un confronto fra l'italiano e l'inglese. In E. M. Thüne & S. Leonardi (Eds.), *Telefonare in diverse lingue. Organizzazione sequenziale, routine e rituali in telefonate di servizio, di emergenza e fàtiche*. FrancoAngeli.

Mushin, I. (2001) *Evidentiality and epistemological stance. Narrative retelling*. John Benjamins.

Nattrass, R., Watermeyer, J., Robson, C., & Penn, C. (2017). Local expertise and landmarks in place reformulations during emergency medical calls. *Journal of Pragmatics, 120*, 73–87.

Neustaedter, C., Jones, B., O'Hara, K., & Sellen, A. (2017). An analysis of next generation 9-1-1: Video calling for emergency situations. *Connections Lab Technical Report 2017-0920-01*, Simon Fraser University.

Neustaedter, C., McGee, J., & Dash, P. (2019). Sharing 9-1-1 video call information between dispatchers and firefighters during everyday emergencies. In *Proceedings of the 2019 on Designing Interactive Systems Conference* (pp. 567–580).

Nordberg, B. (1998). On closings in alarm calls. *Sprak och Stil, 8*, 65–103.

Normark, M. (2002). Sense-making of an emergency call, possibilities and constraints of a computerized case file. *NordiCHI, 10-02*, 81–90.

Normark, M., & Randall, D. (2005). Local expertise at an emergency call centre. In *ECSCW 2005* (pp. 347–366). Springer.

Ong, B. N., Yip, M. P., Feng, S., Calhoun, R., Meischke, H. W., & Tu, S. P. (2012). Barriers and facilitators to using 9-1-1 and emergency medical services in a limited English proficiency Chinese community. *Journal of Immigrant and Minority Health, 14*(2), 307–313.

Orletti, F. (1983). Pratiche di glossa. In F. Orletti (Ed.), *Comunicare nella vita quotidiana* (pp. 77–103). Il Mulino.

Ostermann, A. C., & Harjunpää, K. (2021). OKAY in health helpline calls in Brazilian Portuguese: Managing alignment and progressivity. In E. Betz, A. Deppermann, L. Mondada, & M. L. Sorjonen (Eds.), *OKAY across languages: Toward a comparative approach to its use in talk-in-interaction* (pp. 263–293). John Benjamins.

Osvaldsson, K., Persson-Thunqvist, D., & Cromdal, J. (2013). Comprehension checks, clarifications, and corrections in an emergency call with a nonnative speaker of Swedish. *International Journal of Bilingualism, 17*(2), 205–220.

Palma, E., Antonaci, D., Colì, A., & Cicolini, G. (2014). Analysis of emergency medical services triage and dispatch errors by registered nurses in Italy. *Journal of Emergency Nursing, 40*(5), 476–483.

Palmer, E. C. (1983). Trauma junkies and street work: Occupational behavior of paramedics and emergency medical technicians. *Urban Life, 12*(2), 162–183.

Paoletti, I. (2009). Communication and diagnostic work in medical emergency calls in Italy. *Computer Supported Cooperative Work (CSCW), 18*(2), 229–250.

Paoletti, I. (2012a). Operators managing callers' sense of urgency in calls to the medical emergency number. *Pragmatics, 22*(4), 671–695.

Paoletti, I. (2012b). The issue of conversationally constituted context and localization problems in emergency calls. *Text & Talk, 32*(2), 191–210.

Penn, C., Koole, T., & Nattrass, R. (2017a). When seconds count: A study of communication variables in the opening segment of emergency calls. *Journal of Health Psychology, 22*(10), 1256–1264.

Penn, C., Watermeyer, J., & Nattrass, R. (2017b). Managing language mismatches in emergency calls. *Journal of Health Psychology, 22*(14), 1769–1779.

Perera, N., Riou, M., Ball, S., Birnie, T., Morgan, A., Whiteside, A., Bailey, P., & Finn, J. (2020). The trajectory of repairs in the defibrillator sequence during emergency cardiac arrest calls–balancing progressivity and intersubjectivity. *Communication and Medicine, 17*(2), 150–164.

Perez-Gonzalez, L. (1998). The conversational dynamics of interactional dispute in conflictive calls for emergency assistance: A single case study. In A. Sanchez-Macarro & R. Carter (Eds.), *Linguistic choice across genres: Variation in spoken and written English* (pp. 265–290). John Benjamins.

Pettersson, M. (2001). Talk and visibility: 'One person is out of the car—Did you hear that?'. In S. Björnestad, E. R. Moe, I. A. Mörch, & A. L. Opdahl (Eds.), *Proceedings of the IRIS 24. 11th–14th of August, 2001*, Ulvik, Hardanger, Norway, Iris. 3: 187–200. Retrieved from http://urn.kb.se/resolve?urn=urn:nbn:se:bth-9691

Pettersson, M., & Rouchy, P. (2002). "We don't need an ambulance then!": Technological handling of the unexpected. In *XV World Congress of Sociology, RC.25 Language, Technology and Work*, Brisbane, Australia, 7–13 July.. Retrieved from http://urn.kb.se/resolve?urn=urn:nbn:se:bth-10078

Pichler, H. (2009). The functional and social reality of discourse variants in a northern English dialect: I Don't Know and I Don't Think compared. *Intercultural Pragmatics, 6*(4), 561–596.

Pomerantz, A., & Heritage, J. (2013). Preference. In J. Sidnell & T. Stivers (Eds.), *The handbook of conversation analysis* (pp. 210–229). Wiley-Blackwell.

Potter, J., & Hepburn, A. (2003). "I'm a bit concerned": Early actions and psychological constructions in a child protection helpline. *Research on Language and Social Interaction, 36*(3), 197–240.

Psathas, G. (1979). Organizational features of direction maps. In G. Psaths (Ed.), *Everyday language: Studies in ethnomethodology* (pp. 203–226). Irvington Publishers.

Psathas, G. (1986a). Some sequential structures in direction-giving. *Human Studies, 9*(2), 231–246.

Psathas, G. (1986b). The organization of directions in interaction. *Word, 37*(1–2), 83–91.

Psathas, G. (1987). Finding a place by following directions: A phenomenology of pedestrian and driver wayfinding. *Man-Environment Systems, 17*, 99–103.

Psathas, G. (1990). Direction-giving in interaction. *Reseaux, 8*(1), 183–198.

Psathas, G. (1991). The structure of direction-giving in interaction. In D. Boden & D. Zimmerman (Eds.), *Talk and social structure* (pp. 195–216). Polity Press.

Psathas, G., & Henslin, J. M. (1967). Dispatched orders and the cab driver: A study of locating activities. *Social Problems, 14*(4), 424–443.

Psathas, G., & Kozloff, M. (1976). The structure of directions. *Semiotica, 17*(2), 111–130.

Psathas, G., & Martin, K. (1976). The structure of directions. *Semiotica, 17*(2), 111–130.

Rafaely, D., & Whitehead, K. A. (2020). Extraordinary emergencies: Reproducing moral discourses of the child in institutional interaction. *Pragmatics and Society, 11*(1), 45–69.

Rasmussen, G., Wagner, J., Luke, K. K., & Pavlidou, T. (2002). Language choice in international telephone conversations. In K. K. Luke & T.-S. Pavlidou (Eds.), *Telephone calls: Unity and diversity in conversational structure across languages and cultures* (pp. 111–131). John Benjamins.

Rautiainen, I., Haddington, P., & Kamunen, A. (2022). Local participation framework as a resource among military observer trainees: Interactional episodes between repair initiation and repair solution in critical radio communication. *Journal of Pragmatics, 196*, 67–85.

Raymond, G. (2003). Grammar and social organization: Yes/no interrogatives and the structure of responding. *American Sociological Review, 68*, 939–967.

Raymond, C. W. (2014a). Negotiating entitlement to language: Calling 911 without English. *Language in Society, 43*(1), 33–59.

Raymond, C. W. (2014b). Epistemic brokering in the interpreter-mediated medical visit: Negotiating "patient's side" and "doctor's side" knowledge. *Research on Language and Social Interaction, 47*(4), 426–446.

Raymond, G., & Zimmerman, D. H. (2007). Rights and responsibilities in calls for help: The case of the Mountain Glade Fire. *Research on Language and Social Interaction, 40*(1), 33–61.

Raymond, G., & Zimmerman, D. H. (2016). Closing matters: Alignment and misalignment in sequence and call closings in institutional interaction. *Discourse Studies, 18*(6), 1–34.

Reiter, R. M. (2006). Interactional closeness in service calls to a Montevidean carer service company. *Research on Language and Social Interaction, 39*(1), 7–39.

Relieu, M. (2002). Ouvrir la boîte noire. Identification et localisation dans les conversations mobiles. *Réseaux, 112/113*(2), 20–47.

Relieu, M., Licoppe, C., & Lan Hing Ting, K. (2010). Filmer le travail dans les centres d'appels: le cadrage vidéo et sonore comme mise à l'échelle de l'activité. In G. Vallèry, M.-C. Le Port, & M. Zouinar (Eds.), *Ergonomie, conception de produits et services médiatisés* (pp. 37–55). Presses Universitaires de France.

Riou, M., Ball, S., Williams, T. A., Whiteside, A., O'Halloran, K. L., Bray, J., Perkins, G. D., Smith, K., Cameron, P., Fatovich, D. M., & Inoue, M. (2017). 'Tell me exactly what's happened': When linguistic choices affect the efficiency of emergency calls for cardiac arrest. *Resuscitation, 117*, 58–65.

Riou, M., Ball, S., O'Halloran, K. L., Whiteside, A., Williams, T. A., & Finn, J. (2018a). Hijacking the dispatch protocol: When callers pre-empt their reason-for-the-call in emergency calls about cardiac arrest. *Discourse Studies, 20*(5), 666–687.

Riou, M., Ball, S., Williams, T. A., Whiteside, A., Cameron, P., Fatovich, D. M., Perkins, G. D., Smith, K., Bray, J., Inoue, M., Halloran, K. L., Bailey, P., Brink, D., & Finn, J. (2018b). 'She's sort of breathing': What linguistic factors determine call-taker recognition of agonal breathing in emergency calls for cardiac arrest? *Resuscitation, 122*, 92–98.

Riou, M., Ball, S., Whiteside, A., Gallant, S., Morgan, A., Bailey, P., & Finn, J. (2020). Caller resistance to perform cardio-pulmonary resuscitation in emergency calls for cardiac arrest. *Social Science & Medicine, 256*, 113045.

Robinson, J. D. (2012). Overall structural organization. In J. Sidnell & T. Stivers (Eds.), *The handbook of conversation analysis* (pp. 257–280). Wiley-Blackwell.

Rock, F. (2018). 'Apparently the chap is a bit of a rogue': Upgrading risk in non-emergency telephone calls to the police. *Journal of Applied Linguistics and Professional Practice, 13*(1-3), 276–301.

Rollet, N. (2012). *Analyse conversationnelle des pratiques dans les appels au SAMU-Centre 115: Vers une approche praxéologique d'une forme située 'd'accord'*.. PhD thesis, Université de la Sorbonne nouvelle—Paris III.

Rollet, N. (2013). "D'accord": approche conversationnelle et multimodale d'une forme située dans les appels au Samu-Centre 15. *L'Information grammaticale, 139*, 35–43.

Rollet, N. (2015). Conversations dans l'urgence. *Multitudes, 60*(3), 87–93.

Rønneberg, K., & Svennevig, J. (2010). Declining to help: Rejections in service requests to the police. *Discourse & Communication, 4*(3), 279–305.

Ryle, G. (1966) The world of science and the everyday world. In Id. *Dilemmas* (pp. 68–81). Cambridge University Press.

Sacks, H. (1988). On members' measurement systems. *Research on Language and Social Interaction, 22*(1–4), 45–60.
Sacks, H. (1992). *Lectures on conversation.* Blackwell.
Sacks, H., & Schegloff, E. A. (1979). Two preferences in the organization of reference to persons in conversation and their interaction. In G. Psathas (Ed.), *Everyday language: Studies in ethnomethodology* (pp. 15–21). Irvington Publishers.
Sacks, H., Schegloff, E. A., & Jefferson, G. (1974). A simplest systematics for the organization of turn-taking for conversation. *Language, 50*, 696–735.
Sanders, R. E. (2003). Conversational socializing on marine VHF radio: Adapting laughter and other practices to the technology in use. In P. J. Glenn, C. D. LeBaron, & J. S. Mandelbaum (Eds.), *Studies in language and social interaction* (pp. 309–326). Lawrence Erlbaum Associates.
Schegloff, E. A. (1968). Sequencing in conversational openings. *American Anthropologist, 70*(6), 1075–1095.
Schegloff, E. A. (1972). Notes on a conversational practice: Formulating place. In D. N. Sudnow (Ed.), *Studies in social interaction* (pp. 75–119). Free Press.
Schegloff, E. A. (1979). Identification and recognition in telephone conversation openings. In G. Psathas (Ed.), *Everyday language: Studies in ethnomethodology* (pp. 23–78). Irvington Publishers, Inc.
Schegloff, E. A. (1980). Preliminaries to preliminaries: 'Can I ask you a question?'. *Sociological Inquiry, 50*(3–4), 104–152.
Schegloff, E. A. (1982). Discourse as an interactional achievement: Some uses of "uh huh" and other things that come between sentences. In D. Tannen (Ed.), *Georgetown University roundtable on language and linguistics: Analyzing discourse: Text and talk* (pp. 71–93). Georgetown University Press.
Schegloff, E. A. (1986). The routine as achievement. *Human Studies, 9*(2–3), 111–151.
Schegloff, E. A. (1987). Analyzing single episodes of interaction: An exercise in conversation analysis. *Social Psychology Quarterly, 50*(2), 101–114.
Schegloff, E. A. (1992). Repair after next turn: The last structurally provided defence of intersubjectivity in conversation. *American Journal of Sociology, 97*(5), 1295–1345.
Schegloff, E. A. (2000). On granularity. *Annual Review of Sociology, 26*, 715–720.
Schegloff, E. A. (2002a). Beginnings in the telephone. In J. E. Katz & M. Aakhus (Eds.), *Perpetual contact: Mobile communication, private talk, public performance* (pp. 284–300). Cambridge University Press.
Schegloff, E. A. (2002b). Reflections on research on telephone conversation: Issues of cross-cultural scope and scholarly exchange, interactional import and consequences. In L. Kang Kwong & P. Theodossia-Soula (Eds.), *Telephone calls: Unity and diversity in conversational structure across languages and cultures* (pp. 249–281). John Benjamins.

Schegloff, E. A. (2007). *Sequence organization in interaction: A primer in conversation analysis.* Cambridge University Press.

Schegloff, E. A., & Sacks, H. (1973). Opening up closings. *Semiotica, 8*(4), 289–327.

Schegloff, E. A., Jefferson, G., & Sacks, H. (1977). The preference for self-correction in the organization of repair in conversation. *Language, 53*(2), 361–382.

Scheibman, J. (2000). I dunno: A usage-based account of the phonological reduction of don't in American English conversation. *Journal of Pragmatics, 32*(1), 105–124.

Schuler, S. (2001). Talking community at 911: The centrality of communication in coping with emotional labour. In G. J. Shepered & E. W. Rothenbuhler (Eds.), *Communication and community* (pp. 53–77). Lawrence Erlbaum.

Schutz, A. (1970). *Reflections on the problem of relevance.* Yale University Press.

Scott, J. C. (1998). Thin simplifications and practical knowledge: Metis. In Id., *Seeing like a state* (pp. 309–341). Yale University Press.

Sert, O., & Walsh, S. (2013). The interactional management of claims of insufficient knowledge in English language classrooms. *Language and Education, 27*(6), 542–565.

Sharrock, W. W., & Turner, R. (1978). On a conversational environment for equivocality. In J. N. Schenkein (Ed.), *Studies in the organization of conversational interaction* (pp. 173–197). Academic Press.

Shearing, C. D. (1974). Dial-a-cop: A study of police mobilization. In R. L. Akers & E. Sagarin (Eds.), *Crime prevention and social control* (pp. 77–88). Praeger.

Sidnell, J. (2013). Basic conversation analytic methods. In J. Sidnell & T. Stivers (Eds.), *The handbook of conversation analysis* (pp. 77–99). Willey-Blackwell.

Simmons, J. L. (1974). *Efficient conversation: The talk between pilots and air traffic controllers.* Department of Sociology, University of Colorado. https://files.eric.ed.gov/fulltext/ED088296.pdf

Sorjonen, M.-L. (2021). OKAY in closings and transitions. In E. Betz, A. Deppermann, L. Mondada, & M.-L. Sorjonen (Eds.), *OKAY across languages: Toward a comparative approach to its use in talk-in-interaction* (pp. 94–127). John Benjamins.

Sorjonen, M.-L., Raevaara, L., & Couper-Kuhlen, E. (Eds.). (2017). *Imperative turns at talk: The design of directives in action.* John Benjamins.

Stivers, T., & Robinson, J. D. (2006). A preference for progressivity in interaction. *Language in Society, 35*(3), 367–392.

Stivers, T., & Rossano, F. (2010). Mobilizing response. *Research on Language and Social Interaction, 43*(1), 3–31.

Stivers, T., Rossi, G., & Chalfoun, A. (2022). Ambiguities in action ascription. *Social Forces.* soac021. https://doi.org/10.1093/sf/soac021

Strevens, P. (1984). International maritime English (seaspeak). *Special Language-Fachsprache, 6*(1–2), 2–10.

Suchman, L. (1993). Technologies of accountability: Of lizards and airplanes. In G. Button (Ed.), *Technology in working order: Studies of work, interaction and technology* (pp. 113–126). Routledge.

Suchman, L. (1996). Constituting shared workspaces. In Y. Engestroem & D. Middleton (Eds.), *Cognition and communication at work* (pp. 35–60). Cambridge University Press.

Suchman, L. (1997). Centers of coordination. A case and some themes. In L. Resnick, R. Säljö, C. Pontecorvo, & B. Burge (Eds.), *Discourse, tools and reasoning. Essays on situated cognition* (pp. 41–62). Springer.

Svennevig, J. (2012). On being heard in emergency calls. The development of hostility in a fatal emergency call. *Journal of Pragmatics, 44*(11), 1393–1412.

Svennevig, J., Gerwing, J., Jensen, B. U., & Allison, M. (2019). Pre-empting understanding problems in L1/L2 conversations: Evidence of effectiveness from simulated emergency calls. *Applied Linguistics, 40*(2), 205–227.

Svensson, M., & Hällgren, M. (2018). Sensemaking in sensory deprived settings: The role of non-verbal auditory cues for emergency assessment. *European Management Journal, 36*(3), 306–318.

Szymanski, M. H., Vinkhuyzen, E., Aoki, P. M., & Woodruff, A. (2006). Organizing a remote state of incipient talk: Push-to-talk mobile radio interaction. *Language in Society, 35*(3), 393–418.

Taleghani-Nikazm, C., Betz, E., & Golato, P. (Eds.). (2020). *Mobilizing others: Grammar and lexis within larger activities.* John Benjamins.

ten Have, P. (2002). The notion of member is the heart of the matter: On the role of membership knowledge in ethnomethodological inquiry. *Forum Qualitative Sozialforschung / Forum: Qualitative Social Research, 3*(3). https://doi.org/10.17169/fqs-3.3.834

Tennent, E. (2021). "I'm calling in regard to my son": Entitlement obligation and opportunity to seek help for others. *British Journal of Social Psychology, 60*(3), 870–887.

Tennent, E., & Weatherall, A. (2019). Disclosing violence in calls for help. *Gender and Language, 13*(2), 270–288.

Terasaki, A. (1976). Pre-announcement sequences in conversation. In G. Lerner (Ed.), *Conversation analysis: Studies from the first generation* (pp. 171–223). John Benjamins.

Tjora, A. H. (2000). The technological mediation of the nursing-medical boundary. *Sociology of Health & Illness, 22*(6), 721–741.

Tjora, A. (2004). Maintaining redundancy in the coordination of medical emergencies. In *Proc. of the 2004 ACM Conf. on Computer Supported Cooperative Work.* ACM Press.

Tjora, A. (2009). *Calls for care. Coordination, competence, and computers in medical emergency call centres.* VDM Verlag.

Tracy, K. (1997). Interactional trouble in emergency service requests: A problem of frames. *Research on Language and Social Interaction, 30*(4), 315–343.

Tracy, S. J. (2002). When questioning turns to face threat: An interactional sensitivity in 911 call-taking. *Western Journal of Communication, 66*(2), 129–157.

Tracy, K., & Agne, R. R. (2002). 'I just need to ask somebody some questions': Sensitivities in domestic dispute calls. In J. Cotterill (Ed.), *Language in the legal process* (pp. 75–90). Palgrave.

Tracy, K., & Anderson, D. L. (1999). Relational positioning strategies in police calls: A dilemma. *Discourse Studies, 1*(2), 201–225.

Tracy, K., & Tracy, S. J. (1998a). Rudeness at 911: Reconceptualizing face and face attack. *Human Communication Research, 25*(2), 225–251.

Tracy, S. J., & Tracy, K. (1998b). Emotion labor at 911: A case study and theoretical critique. *Journal of Applied Communication Research, 26*(4), 390–411.

Tsui, A. B. (1991). The pragmatic functions of I don't know. *Text-Interdisciplinary Journal for the Study of Discourse, 11*(4), 607–622.

Tuncer, S. (2016). The effects of video recording on office workers' conduct, and the validity of video data for the study of naturally-occurring interactions. *Forum Qualitative Sozialforschung/Forum: Qualitative Social Research, 17*(3), Art. 7. http://nbn-resolving.de/urn:nbn:de:0114-fqs160373

Vaajala, T., Arminen, I., & De Rycker, A. (2013). Misalignments in Finnish emergency call openings: Legitimacy, asymmetries and multi-tasking as interactional contests. In A. De Rycker & Z. Mohd Don (Eds.), *Discourse and crisis: Critical perspectives* (pp. 131–157). John Benjamins.

Van der Houwen, F., & Sliedrecht, K. Y. (2016). The form and function of formulations: Co-constructing narratives in institutional settings. *Journal of Pragmatics, 105*, 55–58.

Vinkhuyzen, E., & Szymanski, M. H. (2005). Would you like to do it yourself? Service requests and their non-granting responses. In K. Richards & P. Seedhouse (Eds.), *Applying conversation analysis* (pp. 91–106). Palgrave Macmillan.

Vinkhuyzen, E., Whalen, M., & Szymanski, M. (2006). Security, efficiency, and customer service in calls to a financial services organization. *Revue française de linguistique appliquée, 11*(2), 53–68.

Wakin, M. A., & Zimmerman, D. H. (1999). Reduction and specialization in emergency and directory assistance calls. *Research on Language and Social Interaction, 32*(4), 409–437.

Watson, D. R. (1986). Doing the organizations work: An examination of a crisis intervention centre. In S. Fisher & A. D. Todd (Eds.), *Discourse and institutional authority* (pp. 91–120). Ablex.

Weatherall, A. (2011). I don't know as a prepositioned epistemic hedge. *Research on Language & Social Interaction, 44*(4), 317–337.

Weatherall, A., Danby, S., Osvaldsson, K., Cromdal, J., & Emmison, M. (2016). Pranking in children's helpline calls. *Australian Journal of Linguistics, 36*(2), 224–238.

Wennlund, T. K., Kurland, L., Olanders, K., Khoshegir, A., Kamil, H. A., Castrén, M., & Bohm, K. (2022). Emergency medical dispatchers' experiences of managing emergency calls: A qualitative interview study. *BMJ Open, 12*(4), e059803.

Whalen, J. (1995a). Expert systems versus systems for experts: Computer-aided dispatch in public safety communication. In P. Thomas (Ed.), *The social and interactional dimensions of human-computer interfaces* (pp. 161–183). Cambridge University Press.

Whalen, J. (1995b). A technology of order production: Computer-aided dispatch in public safety communication. In P. ten Have & G. Psathas (Eds.), *Situated order. Studies in the social organization of talk and embodied activities* (pp. 187–230). University Press of America.

Whalen, M. R., & Zimmerman, D. H. (1987). Sequential and institutional contexts in calls for help. *Social Psychology Quarterly, 50*(2), 172–185.

Whalen, M. R., & Zimmerman, D. H. (1990). Describing trouble: Practical epistemology in citizen calls to the police. *Language in Society, 19*(4), 465–492.

Whalen, J., & Zimmerman, D. H. (1998). Observations on the display and management of emotion in naturally occurring activities: The case of "hysteria" in calls to 9-1-1. *Social Psychology Quarterly, 61*(2), 141–159.

Whalen, J., & Zimmerman, D. H. (2005). Working a call: Multiparty management and interactional infrastructure in calls for help. In C. D. Baker, M. Emmison, & A. Firth (Eds.), *Calling for help. Language and social interaction in telephone helplines* (pp. 309–345). John Benjamins.

Whalen, J., Zimmerman, D. H., & Whalen, M. (1988). When words fail: A single case analysis. *Social Problems, 35*(4), 335–362.

Wilson, T. P. (1991). Social structure and the sequential organization of interaction. In D. Boden & D. H. Zimmerman (Eds.), *Talk and social structure: Studies in ethnomethodology and conversation analysis* (pp. 22–43). Polity Press.

Wong, B. L. W., & Blandford, A. (2001). Situation awareness and its implications for human–systems interaction. In W. Smith, R. Thomas, et al. (Eds.), *Proc. of the Australian Conf. on computer-human interaction 2001* (pp. 181–186). Ergonomics Society of Australia.

Wong, B. L. W., & Blandford, A. (2002). Analysing ambulance dispatcher decision making: Trialing emergent themes analysis. *Proc. HF2002.* https://discovery.ucl.ac.uk/id/eprint/16628/1/16628.pdf

Woods, C. J., Drew, P., & Leydon, G. M. (2015). Closing calls to a cancer helpline: Expressions of caller satisfaction. *Patient Education and Counselling, 98*(8), 943–953.

Zimmerman, D. H. (1984). Talk and its occasions: The case of calling the police. In D. Schiffrin (Ed.), *Meaning, form, and use in context: Linguistic applications. Georgetown University roundtable on language and linguistics* (pp. 210–228). Georgetown University Press.

Zimmerman, D. H. (1990). Prendre position. In I. Joseph, R. Castel, & J. Cosnier (Eds.), *Le parler frais d'Erving Goffman* (pp. 218–230). Minuit.

Zimmerman, D. H. (1992a). Achieving context: Openings in emergency calls. In G. Watson & R. M. Seiler (Eds.), *Text in context: Contributions to ethnomethodology* (pp. 35–51). Sage.

Zimmerman, D. H. (1992b). The interactional organization of calls for emergency assistance. In P. Drew & J. Heritage (Eds.), *Talk at work: Social interaction in institutional settings* (pp. 418–469). Cambridge University Press.

Zimmerman, D. H. (1998). Identity, context and interaction. In C. Antaki & S. Widdicombe (Eds.), *Identities in talk* (pp. 87–106). Sage.

Index[1]

[1] Note: Page numbers followed by 'n' refer to notes.

G. Fele, *Emergency Communication*, https://doi.org/10.1007/978-3-031-26239-5

The manufacturer's authorised representative in the EU is Springer Nature Customer Service Centre GmbH, Europaplatz 3, 69115 Heidelberg, Germany. If you have any concerns regarding our products, please contact ProductSafety@springernature.com

Printed and bound by CPI Group (UK) Ltd, Croydon, CR0 4YY
01/10/2026
02225894-0001